Children's
Medicines

A JOHNS HOPKINS PRESS HEALTH BOOK

Children's Medicines

WHAT EVERY PARENT, GRANDPARENT,
AND TEACHER NEEDS TO KNOW

Edward A. Bell, PharmD, BCPS

JOHNS HOPKINS UNIVERSITY PRESS
Baltimore

Note to the Reader: This book is not meant to substitute for medical care, and treatment should not be based solely on its contents. Instead, treatment must be developed in a dialogue between the individual and his or her physician. Our book has been written to help with that dialogue.

Drug dosage: The author and publisher have made reasonable efforts to determine that the selection of drugs discussed in this text conform to the practices of the general medical community. The medications described do not necessarily have specific approval by the US Food and Drug Administration for use in the diseases for which they are recommended. In view of ongoing research, changes in governmental regulation, and the constant flow of information relating to drug therapy and drug reactions, the reader is urged to check the package insert of each drug for any change in indications and dosage and for warnings and precautions. This is particularly important when the recommended agent is a new and/or infrequently used drug.

Johns Hopkins University Press
2715 North Charles Street
Baltimore, Maryland 21218-4363
www.press.jhu.edu

An earlier version of this book was published as *A Parent's Guide to Children's Medicines* (© 2012 Edward A. Bell).

Library of Congress Cataloging-in-Publication Data
Names: Bell, Edward A., 1959– author.
Title: Children's medicines : what every parent, grandparent, and teacher needs to know / Edward A. Bell, PharmD, BCPS.
Description: Baltimore : Johns Hopkins University Press, 2017. | Includes bibliographical references and index.
Identifiers: LCCN 2017007354| ISBN 9781421423746 (hardcover : alk. paper) | ISBN 142142374X (hardcover : alk. paper) | ISBN 9781421423753 (pbk. : alk. paper) | ISBN 1421423758 (pbk. : alk. paper) | ISBN 9781421423760 (electronic) | ISBN 1421423766 (electronic)
Subjects: LCSH: Pediatric pharmacology—Popular works. | Drugs—Popular works.
Classification: LCC RJ560 .B44 2017 | DDC 615.1083—dc23
   LC record available at https://lccn.loc.gov/2017007354

A catalog record for this book is available from the British Library.

Special discounts are available for bulk purchases of this book. For more information, please contact Special Sales at 410-516-6936 or specialsales@press.jhu.edu.

Johns Hopkins University Press uses environmentally friendly book materials, including recycled text paper that is composed of at least 30 percent post-consumer waste, whenever possible.

Contents

Preface

Parents and other caregivers have many decisions to make on behalf of their children. A decision that comes up often, especially early in childhood or for children who have chronic illnesses, is whether the child would benefit from a medicine—a prescription medicine, an over-the-counter medicine product, or perhaps an alternative therapy, such as an herbal medicine. Most often, these medicines are recommended by your child's pediatrician or family doctor, a nurse practitioner provider, or another health care provider. At other times, you may be wondering whether to treat your child with an over-the-counter product or an alternative medicine. Are these medicines safe for your infant or child? Are they likely to be effective and to help your child? When is it best *not* to give a medicine to your child? Another common question is about pediatric vaccines: are they safe, and are they still necessary? All parents share these concerns.

With so much medical information easily available to the public, whether by drug advertisements on television or Internet sites, answering these questions to your own satisfaction can be a daunting job. It is easy for parents to get confused when faced with these decisions and the abundance of sometimes conflicting available information. It is my hope that this book will help you answer some of these questions and assist you in feeling more comfortable making decisions on the role and use of medicines and other therapies for your child and family. There are many good books written by pediatricians that are currently available on pediatric health and medical topics. *Children's Medicines* is not meant to replace these books—it can supplement them by providing additional drug therapy information. The information in this book is presented and described in a pharmacy frame of reference—the subjects discussed include practical points relating to questions about medicines to ask your pediatrician and pharmacist, and how to most appropriately use many specific pediatric prescription and over-the-counter drug products to improve your child's health.

Children's Medicines discusses the science behind safe and effective medicine use in infants, children, and adolescents, and additionally gives practical advice and recommendations on how best to give medicines to your child. I have prepared this book as a pediatric pharmacist, from experiences gained in hospital and clinic settings, and as a university professor and a parent. The topics and information contained in this book I have frequently researched in preparation for the classes on pediatric drug therapy I teach to pharmacy students, and for the regularly published drug therapy column that I write for a national pediatric medical news journal. It is my intent to provide you with scientifically up-to-date and accurate information on medicines and alternative therapy products that may be helpful to your family's health and well-being. Practical tips and recommendations are additionally presented that can help you choose, obtain, and administer the most appropriate and best medicine for your family.

This book would not have been possible without the support and advice from the following, whom I thank:

My wife and children, for their love and support.

The College of Pharmacy and Health Sciences of Drake University, for granting me sabbatical leave and the time to write this book.

The health care professionals of Blank Children's Hospital and Clinics.

The following individuals, for providing valuable advice and content review:

Dr. Wendi Harris, pediatrician reviewer, Clive, Iowa

Dr. Ken Cheyne, pediatrician reviewer, Clive, Iowa

Dr. Lynne Maxwell, Philadelphia, Pennsylvania

The publishing staff of Johns Hopkins University Press.

Children's
Medicines

1

The Science of Medicines for Children

"Children are not small adults" and children are "therapeutic orphans." These two phrases, coined over 50 years ago, still ring true today in regard to the use of medications in pediatric medicine. When treating medical conditions, physicians know that infants, young children, and even adolescents may not respond the same way as an adult would to an administered medication, and often the safety and efficacy of a drug have not been tested in this population.

Years ago, doses of medicines given to infants and children were often crudely estimated (extrapolated) by comparing them to an adult medicine dose and a typical adult's weight or body size. For some medicines, this still occurs today. For example, a 3-year-old child's weight may be approximately 25 percent of a typical adult's weight, and thus the child is given 25 percent of the adult dose of a medicine. Over the past 50+ years, we have learned much more about how medicines behave, or function, differently in an infant or child's body, as compared to an adult's, and how ineffective or dangerous medicine dose extrapolation can be. Drug functioning refers to how medicines are absorbed, distributed, metabolized, and excreted within and from the body. Drug functioning also refers to the drug's mechanism of action, to yield its therapeutic benefits (for example, relief of symptoms or cure of an infection).

In this chapter, I discuss the underlying principles of how medicines are studied and evaluated in infants and children; common problems (and solutions) parents face when choosing and administering medicines; examples of medicines that should *not* be given to infants or children; and other factors that relate to safe and effective medicine use. In the rest of the book, I discuss the treatment of common pediatric medical problems, vaccines, and the "art" of medicine use in infants and children, including tips for administering medicines to infants and young children. After all, a safe and effective medicine will not be of much help if your child will not take it.

This information will help caregivers understand how medications function in children (differently from in an adult) and what medical conditions can be treated with prescription and over-the-counter (OTC) medications, as well as which medications are potentially dangerous for a child. With this understanding, parents, grandparents, and other caregivers will be better able to decide when medicine therapy can be a safe and effective choice to improve a child's health.

Testing Medicine in the Pediatric Population

One of the major challenges pediatric health care professionals, such as myself, frequently face is the lack of approval of medicines in the pediatric population. By definition, the pediatric population includes ages less than 18 years. "Approval" is not an accurate word for this topic, but it is commonly used. The United States government agency that regulates the use (that is, the manufacturing, safety, and advertising) of medicines is the Food and Drug Administration (FDA). The FDA strives to ensure that medicinal products are safe and effective when used according to the drug product's labeling.

A medicine's label is the official information included with the product bottle or packaging, and it describes the medicine's dosage, adverse effects, contraindications, and interactions, among other important information. Health care professionals must review this information prior to prescribing or dispensing the medication to ensure that the medicine is used appropriately for a specific patient. This also applies to a parent or other caregiver when an OTC medicine is given to an infant or child: the parent, grandparent, daycare provider, or school nurse should read and understand the medicine product's labeling or information prior to administering it to the child.

The product information that accompanies prescription medicines is written in medical language, not in language designed for the general public. These information sheets are included with the medicine by the manufacturer. Labeling of an OTC product includes informational wording on the product package and bottle—this is written for the public. So, the FDA does not "approve" the specific use of medicines—they approve medicines' labeling, and it is then incumbent upon health care professionals, and consumers (parents), to ensure that medicines are used appropriately. This does not always occur, however. So it is more accurate to say that a medicine is "labeled" for specific uses or, for purposes of this discussion, a medicine is labeled for use in specific ages.

Unfortunately, most medicines—more than 50 percent of them—are *not* labeled for use in the pediatric population. Why? Because the medicines have not been studied or tested in this population. Studying and testing medicines in the pediatric population is considerably more difficult for a drug manufacturer; generally because it is more expensive and it is difficult to enroll study subjects (infants or small children). Unless a medicine is likely to be prescribed frequently in the pediatric population, a drug manufacturer is unlikely to test and study its drug in this population. Thus, most medicines are "labeled" for use only in adults. When a new medicine is labeled for adult use only by the FDA, we do not know the pediatric dose, nor do we know if the medicine is even safe or effective to use in the pediatric population. We know that some medicines can have different, or more severe, adverse effects or toxicities in infants and children, as compared to in adults (see the following pages for several examples). The best means to determine the safety and efficacy of medicines in infants and children is to formally test and study them in these ages.

Every single day, medicines are prescribed to infants and children that are not labeled for use at their age. This is referred to as "off-label" use and, fortunately, most of the time, significant adverse effects do not occur. However, the potential for significant adverse effects or lack of efficacy is greater when a medicine is used off-label in pediatrics, and thus medical professionals would prefer that all medicines prescribed for infants and children be labeled for their ages.

Although improvements are still needed, pediatric drug labeling —formally testing and studying medicines in the pediatric population—has advanced during the past 25 years. Two major legislative acts have contributed to this—the Best Pharmaceuticals for Children Act (BPCA) and the Pediatric Research Equity Act (PREA). In 2012, the BPCA and the PREA were reauthorized under the FDA Safety and Innovation Act. These legislations have used both a carrot and a stick approach (incentives and requirements) to entice pharmaceutical manufacturers to formally test and label more drug products for use in the pediatric population. If a medicine is determined to have significant beneficial use for infants and children, then the manufacturer is required to formally study and test it in infants and children. For other medicines in specified circumstances, a manufacturer may voluntarily study their medicine in the pediatric population in return for certain financial incentives, such as extended marketing exclusivities.

One recently published study found that between 1998 and 2012 the FDA granted new pediatric labeling information for more than 170 medicines. Collectively, implementation of BPCA and PREA has resulted in more than 500 pediatric drug labeling changes, a significant step toward a greater availability of drug information for health care professionals. Significantly, some medicines studied in the pediatric population turned out to *not be* effective for treatment of specific medical problems in infants or children—even when those medications had been shown to be effective for the same condition in adults.

The differences in how medicines function in, and how diseases affect, the pediatric versus the adult population explains why we say that "children are not small adults." The physiologic and medical differences between children and adults underlie certain specific disease states, such as some types of cancer. Also, medicines behave or function differently in an infant or child's body as compared to an adult's body. Although the pediatric population includes ages younger than 18 years, some medicines are labeled for use in specific pediatric subgroups. For example, it is not uncommon for some medicines to be labeled for use at 12 years of age and older, and in adults. While a 12-year-old boy or girl is considered a pediatric patient, the dose and adverse effects of many medicines at this age may not differ significantly from that of an adult. In general, the younger the pediatric patient, the more likely a medicine's dose, adverse effects, contraindications, and so on will differ from that of an adult, and thus the more we need information from pediatric testing. How a medicine behaves or functions in a 1-year-old infant male can significantly differ from how it behaves or functions in a 15-year-old adolescent male, although both of these males are classified as belonging within the pediatric population. Neonates—infants younger than 1 month of age—demonstrate even greater differences in how medicines function, and for most medicines, we have very little information on how to best use medicines safely and effectively in newborn infants.

It is also important to note that although most medicines are not formally FDA age labeled for use in infants and children, we have accumulated many years of pediatric clinical experience for some of them. This experience is often described and published in medical journals. Your child's physician, prescriber, or pharmacist likely subscribes to some of these medical journals. For example, albuterol is a commonly used medicine to treat breathing problems, such as asthma, in infants and children. Albuterol is given as a metered dose inhaler or as a solution in a nebulizer. Albuterol inhalers such as Ventolin HFA or Proair HFA are labeled for use in children 4 years of age and older, and albuterol nebulizer solutions are labeled for use at 2 years of age and older. However, because breathing difficulties occur so often in infants and young children, albuterol is commonly given to infants less than 2 years of age, and when used appropriately (the correct dose and frequency) for these young patients, it is safe and effective. Why is a medicine such as albuterol not labeled for use in these young ages if it is commonly used? Obtaining FDA age labeling would require the pharmaceutical manufacturer to submit thousands of pages of data from formal drug testing and studies in these ages, and because this is expensive and difficult, it is not done.

When we have the practical experience of many years of safe and effective clinical use of the medicine in these age groups, we are not quite as concerned with FDA age labeling, although it would certainly be welcomed. We are most concerned when giving new medicines, or medicines with which we have very little pediatric clinical experience, to infants and children that are not age labeled by the FDA. It is also important to note that some medicines include warnings or contraindications that are more likely to have significant adverse effects or toxicities when given to infants or children. These medicines should rarely, or never, be given to infants and children. This distinction—prescribing a medicine that does not have pediatric FDA labeling versus giving a medicine that is contraindicated or more likely to cause harm to an infant or child—is important to understand.

How should you, as a parent or other caregiver, evaluate information about labeling? First off, you should ask your child's physician or nurse practitioner if the prescribed medicine is labeled for use at your child's age. If the medicine is not labeled at this age, ask how much clinical experience the medical community has had using this medicine in infants or children. If the medicine is not age labeled, ask your pediatrician if it is likely to be effective and safe for treating your child's illness.

TOO OFTEN in our society, it is only when a bad event occurs that we act to improve our laws and public safety. Such an event occurred in 1937, prompting initiation and establishment of our current federal laws regulating drug safety.

Sulfanilamide, an antibiotic used to treat streptococcal (strep) throat infections, was in use in tablet and powder forms. However, a need developed to have sulfanilamide available in liquid form as well, likely to treat children. The pharmaceutical manufacturer developed a liquid dosage form by dissolving sulfanilamide in diethylene glycol, and it was formulated to be pleasing in appearance, fragrance, and taste. Unfortunately, this new drug solution was not tested for toxicity and safety, as this was not required by law at that time. Diethylene glycol is a component of antifreeze products and is toxic.

This new sulfanilamide solution was shipped throughout the United States, resulting in the deaths of 107 people, mostly children. This tragic experience demonstrated the necessity for drug safety laws and prompted the establishment of the Federal Food, Drug, and Cosmetic Act (FDC) of 1938. The FDC authorized numerous new laws and regulations controlling drug and food safety and required that new medicines demonstrate safety before they could be marketed and sold.

In 1962, severe pediatric drug toxicity again prompted the establishment of important new drug safety laws and regulations. Thalidomide, a medicine used as an adult sedative in Europe, was administered to pregnant women to treat severe morning sickness. Unfortunately, it was found to be highly teratogenic (causing birth defects) when taken during pregnancy, resulting in severe birth defects in many thousands of babies. In the United States, the FDA became aware of this danger and passed the Kefauver-Harris Drug Amendments, establishing laws requiring medicines to be proven effective as well as safe prior to marketing and sale.

Medicines Behave Differently in Infants and Children as Compared to Adults

As discussed in the previous section, all medicines behave, or function, differently in infants and children as compared to in adults. The younger the infant or child, the more important these differences become. As parents know, the bodies and behavior of infants and children change quite rapidly during childhood. For example, a healthy infant's weight will double at about age 6 months, triple at 12 months, and quadruple at 24 months. I am certainly glad that my weight does not double in 6 months!

When a medicine's pharmacology is reviewed, four major areas are discussed:

- Absorption
- Distribution
- Metabolism
- Excretion

Collectively they are known by the acronym ADME.

Most medicines function inside the body and must be absorbed into the blood and then distributed throughout the body to their site of action. Some medicines function topically—they are applied to the skin to treat conditions such as acne or to protect the skin from damage, for example, from the sun. Even when a medicine is applied to the skin, some of the medicine is absorbed and enters the bloodstream. Differences in skin characteristics (for example, thickness, hydration status) between an infant, older child, and adult can be very important and can increase a medicine's adverse effects. For example, topical corticosteroid (anti-inflammatory) creams or ointments are commonly used to treat inflammatory diaper rash in infants. Numerous different corticosteroid medicines are available, and they differ primarily in their potency, or strength. Hydrocortisone is one of the least potent topical corticosteroids, and beclomethasone is a more potent topical corticosteroid.

Since infants characteristically have thinner, more hydrated skin, caution should be used in applying more potent corticosteroids like beclomethasone. If too much of a potent corticosteroid is absorbed through the skin, severe adverse effects may occur. Case reports describing this scenario have been published in medical journals. If a physician diagnoses an infant with inflammatory diaper rash, a low potency topical corticosteroid cream or ointment, such as hydrocortisone, may be indicated. The parent should apply only a thin layer of the corticosteroid to the affected skin, and when used appropriately, it is likely to be safe and effective.

Most medicines are given to infants and children orally, and physiologic differences among infants, children, and adults can affect oral medicine absorption. These differences include the pH (acidity) of the stomach and how quickly swallowed medicines move through the stomach and intestines (medicines are absorbed into the blood from the intestinal tract), among others. These differences, affecting the amount and rate at which medicines are absorbed into the blood to reach their site of action, can result in important clinical alterations in how we use medicines in the pediatric population. Once a medicine is absorbed into the blood, it distributes throughout the body. A medicine's chemical characteristics and physiologic factors affect how widely it distributes, and to what areas of the body. The main physiologic factors include body water content and proteins in the blood. A healthy infant born at term gestation (≥ 37 weeks) is composed of approximately 75 percent water; in comparison, an adult is 55 to 60 percent water. As the amount of body water decreases in infancy, body fat increases. Medicines can display important chemical differences in their attraction for water (hydrophilic) or fat (lipophilic), and these characteristics affect how widely the medicine distributes throughout the body (known as the drug's volume of distribution). Some medicines are transported in the blood by attaching to blood proteins, namely albumin. Differences in the quantity and quality of albumin and other blood proteins in infants, children, and adults can affect how safe and effective a medicine is. Some medicines that extensively bind to albumin, such as the commonly used antibiotic Rocephin, can cause levels of bilirubin (a breakdown product of red blood cells) to dangerously increase in newborn infants, resulting in jaundice. This adverse effect is less likely to occur in older infants, children, and adults.

Medicines are removed from our bodies primarily by the liver and kidneys. The liver additionally functions to metabolize many chemicals that our bodies naturally produce, and chemicals and medicines that are introduced into our bodies. Some medicines are not active in the body until they are metabolized by the liver to an active form. Within the liver are numerous types of specific enzymes that metabolize medicines and these natural chemicals. At birth, many of these metabolizing enzymes are not fully mature, and are much less active. They mature, or become active, at different rates, with some drug-metabolizing systems not fully maturing until 3 to 5 years of age, or even until the adolescent years for others.

Well-known examples of the severe consequences of administering medicines that have not been tested or studied in infants and children to that population include the antibiotic chloramphenicol and the drug product preservative benzyl alcohol. When given to young infants, chloramphenicol and benzyl alcohol can result in severe adverse effects, including death, known as "gray baby syndrome" for chloramphenicol and the "gasping syndrome" for benzyl alcohol. Conversely, the efficiency of other drug metabolizing systems in the liver, once fully matured, are significantly greater in young children as opposed to adults. This results in the need for larger weight-based doses of some medicines as compared to adults.

The kidneys are also responsible for eliminating many medicines from the body. At birth, a healthy infant's kidneys function well enough to eliminate waste products in urine. However, this functioning efficiency is decreased as compared to older children and adults, and it matures at approximately 1 year of age. This difference becomes important for medicines that are eliminated from the body primarily through the kidneys. If the frequency of dosing is not adjusted for the infant's age, it can lead to increased drug adverse effects or toxicity. Similar to drug elimination by the liver, as drug elimination by the kidneys matures in young children, it may become even more efficient than in adults, requiring some medicines to be given more frequently than to an adult.

Thus, as infants and children grow, their bodies undergo significant changes, and these changes affect how we use medicines, including dosing, adverse effects, and the potential for severe toxicity. Testing and studying medicines in the pediatric population is the best means to improve their safe and effective use.

OVER-THE-COUNTER medicines for coughs and colds have historically been commonly used in pediatrics. In 2008, the FDA recommended that they not be given to children under 4 years of age, and the FDA is continuing to review if this recommendation should extend to children up to 11 years of age. The reasons for this recommendation represent a good example of the information discussed in this chapter, and serve to highlight the potential dangers when medicines are used that have not been tested and demonstrated to be safe and effective in infants and children.

The numerous different active ingredients in cough and cold medicine products have been "generally recognized as safe and effective" for use in adults. Since the 1970s, the FDA has known that information demonstrating their safety and effectiveness in infants and children was essentially nonexistent. However, as they were commonly used in the pediatric population, in 1974 the FDA asked a panel of seven physicians to develop cough and cold medicine product dosing guidelines for pediatric use. Their dosing recommendations included ages younger than 2 years (consult a physician); ages 2 to 5 years (give one-quarter

(*continued*)

of an adult dose); and ages 6 to 11 years (give one-half of an adult dose).

These dosing guidelines were not based upon safety and efficacy studies but were extrapolated from doses appropriate for adults, which flies in the face of all the information discussed above and highlights the dangers of giving untested medicines to infants and children. You may wonder why cough and cold medicines would be effective in adults but not children. The answer is complex, but likely relates to how differently medicines function in infants and children, and how medical conditions, such as coughs and colds, differ physiologically between the pediatric and adult populations.

More recently, several well-done clinical studies evaluating cough and cold medicines in the young pediatric population have been published and have shown that they are not effective. As well, case reports of the dangers of these products when given to infants and young children have been published, with more than 100 deaths documented. Unfortunately, it becomes very easy for parents to give excessive doses of these medicines, resulting in toxicity, as small doses are difficult to accurately measure, and as they are not effective, the idea that "more is better" leads some parents to give more of the ineffective medication. See chapter 3 for more about treating coughs and colds in infants and children.

Medicine's Adverse Effects Can Differ in Pediatrics

Further descriptions and explanations of how medicines differ in the pediatric population relate to the unique adverse effects some medicines produce in infants and children. Most parents are aware that children should not receive aspirin (a contraindication) when treating fever in infants and children, as aspirin use can result in severe liver and brain injury, and death, known as Reye's syndrome. Reye's syndrome is more likely to occur when aspirin is given to a child with a viral infection, such as influenza. In 1986 the FDA recommended that aspirin and chemically similar medicines (salicylates) not be given to children 18 years of age and younger when treating illnesses with fever. Aspirin can be cautiously used in some children when treating other medical conditions, such as Kawasaki disease, and should only be given when recommended by a physician.

Tetracycline is an older antibiotic that still has many uses to treat bacterial infections. Tetracycline should not be given to children less than 8 years of age, however, as it can bind with calcium in teeth and bones, resulting in an ugly gray staining of teeth and decreased bone growth. Antihistamines are commonly given to children and adults to treat a variety of symptoms, most notably allergic conditions. Older antihistamines, such as diphenhydramine (for example, Benadryl), can commonly cause sedation or drowsiness. Young children given these older antihistamines can also develop paradoxical adverse reactions, resulting in excitability, tremors, convulsions, or hallucinations. These adverse reactions are significantly less likely to occur in children given newer antihistamines, such as cetirizine (for example, Zyrtec) or loratadine (for example, Claritin).

Conversely, adverse effects from some medicines are *less* likely to occur in children as compared to adults. Ibuprofen (sold under the common trade names Motrin and Advil) and other nonsteroidal anti-inflammatory drugs (NSAIDs) are commonly given to children and adults to treat fever, pain, and various inflammatory conditions. A feared and relatively common adverse effect of ibuprofen and other NSAID use in adults is bleeding from the intestinal tract, such as from an ulcer. Fortunately, this adverse effect rarely occurs in children. Isoniazid is an antibiotic used to treat tuberculosis and other infections and may cause severe inflammation of the liver in adults. This is another example where the medicine's adverse effect is significantly less likely to occur in children.

From an understanding of how medicines are absorbed, distributed, metabolized, and eliminated from the body, and their potential for unique adverse effects, comes a major principle: *in many ways, medicines behave and function differently in infants and children as compared to in adults.* Keep this principle in mind when speaking with your child's physician, pharmacist, and other health care providers and when choosing medicine therapies for your child. Recently enacted regulations requiring more medicines to be tested in children have improved our knowledge of how to use medicines safely and effectively in the pediatric population. Many medicines, however, remain inadequately studied in infants and children, and so the parent and the health care providers need to work together to be informed and choose wisely when it comes to a child's medications.

Summary Points for Parents

- Many medicines are not tested and studied in the pediatric population, although new laws and regulations now require more medicines to be tested and studied in infants and children prior to their being marketed and made available to the public.

- Many differences exist between how medicines function and distribute in infants, children, and adults. These differences affect medicine effectiveness and safety.

- Some medicines can result in more adverse effects in children than in adults.

- Knowledge of these differences, as well as appreciation for how medicines are tested in children, can aid parents when choosing and discussing medicine therapies with their child's physician, pharmacist, and other health care professionals.

2

The Art and Practicality of Giving Medicine to Children

As parents of sick children know, it is not always easy to measure out exact liquid medication doses. The younger the child, the harder it can be to give medicine and to judge if the medicine is helping. A number of potential problems can increase the difficulty of administering accurate doses of medicine to infants and children.

In this chapter I describe the best ways to give medications to infants and children, including medicine doses in tablet, capsule, and liquid form. I also explain how typical administration problems come about, and I suggest ways to avoid these problems. Common mistakes with medications may not always result in harm to a child, but significant adverse effects and harm from medication mistakes have been shown and are well known to have occurred. Researchers have evaluated many of these topics, and the results of their studies are discussed here.

Common Mistakes and Problems Parents and Other Caregivers Face

Many published studies have shown that it is easy for parents to make mistakes when giving prescription and over-the-counter (OTC) medicines to their children. For example, in some studies parents were given a common pediatric medicine bottle, such as liquid antibiotics or liquid acetaminophen (Tylenol), and were asked to calculate a dose for their child. Study parents were given their child's current weight and were also asked to measure the calculated dose with their choice of different dosing devices. (I'll say more about these studies and their results in the following pages.)

All of the common parental mistakes discussed in this chapter can be easily avoided when parents know what the potential problems are. By following several simple rules caregivers can avoid these pitfalls. Common mistakes include:

- not reading the medication bottle instructions or label properly,
- not accurately measuring doses of liquid medicines,
- determining a child's dose by age and not by weight,
- giving too many medicines at one time (over-medicating), and
- not finishing the full amount of a prescribed medicine.

Some of these medicine mistake "categories," such as not reading the medicine label or instructions carefully, happen when adults give themselves medicine as well. It can be easy to inaccurately administer an OTC or prescription medication to your child if you do not read the label on the bottle and product packaging. Unfortunately, the ability to buy an OTC medication without speaking with a physician or pharmacist makes this too easy to do.

Let's take these points one at a time.

Not Knowing Your Child's Weight

As your child rapidly grows, his or her weight increases, meaning your child needs a higher dose than you may have previously administered. Weights of infants and children increase significantly in the first few years of life. As mentioned in chapter 1, the weight of a healthy infant can double at 6 months, triple at 12 months, and quadruple at 24 months of age. Another issue connected to weight is that medicines come in different concentrations. You might try a different liquid product that has a better flavor, and a different concentration, and consequently you give an incorrect dose based on your child's weight.

Basing the Dose on Age Rather Than Weight

Many OTC medication products list medication dose ranges for specific ages (for example, "for ages 4–6 years, give X mg"), and because parents don't always know their child's current weight, it is easy to rely on the age range on the product label. But your child's weight may differ from the age range listed on the product. While it may seem straightforward to rely on your child's age, determining a medication dose based specifically on your infant's or child's current *weight* is more accurate, and is most likely to help your child, without resulting in adverse effects.

Inaccuracy in Determining and Measuring Doses of Liquid Medicine

This is probably the most common mistake parents make, and the mistake most closely studied by researchers. It is described in more detail in the following pages.

Giving Too Many Medicines, or Over-Medicating, Your Child

Healthy infants and children are frequently ill with colds and other common maladies, often more so than adults, and pharmaceutical manufacturers market many OTC products to treat these illnesses. Many of these products should not be used in children, as they have not been proven to be safe and effective in infants and children. Yet, it is tempting to try them, and as they are often not effective, it becomes easy to try giving more. In this case, more is *not* better!

Not Administering All of the Medicine as Prescribed

The best example of this common mistake relates to antibiotics. Antibiotics typically begin to help within 72 hours, and by 5 days or so, your child often seems significantly improved. But generally

Table 2.1 Information points to discuss with your child's doctor and pharmacist about your child's medicine

NAME OF THE MEDICINE*
> Most drugs have two names—a trade name and a generic name (for example—Tylenol [trade] is acetaminophen [generic]). Ask if the prescribed medicine is available in a generic form.

DOSE
- For liquid medicines
  - What are the volume (mL) dose and the mg dose? (for example, amoxicillin liquid 5 mL usually is equivalent to 400 mg).
- For tablets and capsules
  - How many mg are in one tablet or capsule?
  - How many tablets or capsules should I give each day?

DOSING SCHEDULE
- How many times a day should I give the medicine?
- If dosing once a day, can I give the medicine at any time during the day?
- Can the medicine be given with meals?
- Is the medicine to be given as needed only, or scheduled every day?

DURATION
- How long should I give the medicine?
  - Some pediatric medicines are given for short durations (for example, antibiotics).
  - Other medicines (for example, those for a chronic condition like asthma) are taken for longer durations.

BENEFITS TO YOUR CHILD
- How will the medicine help my child?
- What should I look for to be sure it is helping?
- How long will it take until the medicine begins to help?

MISSED DOSES
- If I miss a dose, what should I do?

ADVERSE EFFECTS
- What are the most common adverse effects of the medicine?
- What should I do if adverse effects occur?
- What can I do to decrease adverse effects?
- Are there any rare but serious adverse effects?

STORAGE
- For liquid medicine
  - Should it be stored at room temperature, in the refrigerator, or does it not matter?
- Can the medicine be divided into different, but labeled, containers for use at school and home?
- It is best not to store medicine in nonpharmacy-labeled bottles. If it is misplaced or lost, whoever finds it may not know what medicine it is.

---

* Keep a list of your child's medicines (name, dose, and schedule) in your cell phone "Notes" or on a piece of paper you carry.

antibiotics are prescribed for a course of 10 or more days. It becomes tempting to stop the antibiotic and save it for your child's next fever or illness, even though this antibiotic was likely prescribed for longer.

Your Child's New Medicine: What to Discuss with Your Pediatrician and Pharmacist

When you are in the pediatrician's office, or at the pharmacy picking up your child's medicine, it is helpful to have in mind what information you should seek about your child's new medicine. This information, listed in table 2.1, is important for all medications. Your child's pediatrician and pharmacist will almost certainly talk with you about the specific medication dose and how often the dose should be given. Some of the other points—such as proper storage—may or may not be raised.

When I have senior pharmacy students with me in the pediatric clinic I attend, I give them an index card containing the discussion points listed in table 2.1 so they can use it as a guide when counseling patients on newly prescribed medicines. I have seen many instances of parents either not being given all of this information, or of not quite understanding how to use the information they received. Even with the best of intentions, parents sometimes forget what they have been told (it's easy to do when you are concerned about a sick child). As a consequence of not having information, not understanding information, or forgetting information, a parent may not administer a medication correctly and it will not help as much as it would have if it had been given properly.

Consider these points when discussing your child's medicine with your pediatrician or pharmacist.

Dosing Schedule

For many medications, the time of day it is given, or the spacing of doses (how many hours pass between doses), is not critical. What's important with these medications is that all of the daily doses are indeed given, and that the dosing schedule is the best fit for you and your child's daily routine. For medications prescribed once daily, it may not matter if the medication is given in the morning, at noon, or at bedtime. For some medications, however, it does matter, so ask about this. Some medications may cause drowsiness or, alternatively, may be somewhat stimulating; these properties of the medication may affect what time of day you give the medicine (give at bedtime, or in the morning, respectively).

Morning is often a hectic time for many school-aged children or adolescents, so giving medicine in the afternoon or evening may work better with their schedules. When medications are prescribed to be given three times a day to school-aged children, ask if the medicine can be administered before school, after school, and in the evening, instead of at school, which may be difficult to arrange.

For medications prescribed "every 8 hours" or "every 12 hours," and so on, the timing is usually not critically important. For example, if the second daily dose is given 9 to 10 hours, instead of 12 hours, after the first dose, this likely will not affect the medication's benefit or have any adverse effects for your child. However, ask the doctor or pharmacist about how important the schedule is, to be sure. For some medications, such as those for treating seizure disorders, dose schedule timing may be more important. I've seen many families where medicine doses were missed because they could not strictly adhere to this type of schedule, and the families were concerned about giving doses too close or too far apart. It's also important to be consistent—strive to give the medicine at approximately the same time each day, once you settle on a good schedule for you and your child.

Benefits to Your Child

Some medicines work quickly, within 1 hour, to help your child feel better. Good examples are medications for fever and pain, such as acetaminophen (Tylenol) and ibuprofen (Motrin, Advil). Other medicines may not begin to significantly help your child for 1 to 2 weeks, or longer. Examples include many antidepressant medications, such as fluoxetine (Prozac).

It is important to understand how you or your child will know if the medicine is helping. Don't hesitate to ask your pediatrician or pharmacist, "How will I know if the medicine is helping my child? What should I look for?" I have spoken with adolescents who had been prescribed antidepressants but had stopped taking them because they did not know if they were making a difference. After we talked about how they might not recognize that the medication was helping them, they realized the medicine was beneficial.

Missed Doses

Everyone, including me, forgets a dose of his or her medicine at times. What should you do once you realize that you missed a dose of your child's medicine? This depends upon the specific medicine and how long it has been since the scheduled time of the dose. For many medications, even if several hours or more have passed since the scheduled time, it is better to give the missed dose instead of skipping it. This is not true for all medications, however, so ask what to do if a dose is missed. Many patients have told me over the years that they skipped doses completely because they missed their normal scheduled time. If this happens 2 or 3 days each week, which can be easy to do, the result may be that the medicine provides much less benefit.

Adverse Effects

One aspect of giving medicine to children that concerns many parents is a medicine's adverse effects. This is certainly understandable. When you leave the pediatrician's office or the pharmacy, you should have no lingering or unanswered concerns about your child's medicine. *All* medications have potential to cause adverse effects. Adverse effects that nearly all oral medications may cause include nausea, vomiting, diarrhea, headache, or drowsiness/dizziness. Some of these effects may be minimized by, for example, giving some medications with meals (note, though, that some medications must *not* be taken with food).

A word of caution about the printed information you may receive at the pharmacy along with your child's new medicine, or what you read online about a medicine. The adverse effects listed in the medication's labeling (see chapter 1 for more on medication labeling) may not necessarily occur with your child. These listed adverse effects, which typically are many, occurred when the medication was studied and tested, and may or may not have directly resulted from the medication. As described in table 2.1, ask what adverse effects commonly occur with your child's medicine and what you can to do minimize or prevent them. Ask what more serious adverse effects may occur and which adverse effects make it necessary to stop the medicine or return to your pediatrician's office.

Some parents state that they are concerned about a medication's "toxicities." This is not the same as a medication's adverse effects, or side effects. *Adverse effects* of a medication are unwanted and unintended effects of the medication. For example, antibiotics commonly produce nausea or loose stools—unwanted effects. Adverse effects can occur with just one dose of a medication—they can be mild or severe, common or uncommon, and predictable or unpredictable. *Toxicity* refers to the effects that occur from a medication dose that is greater than the normal therapeutic dosing range (the amount of medication normally given to treat a medical condition). Acetaminophen (Tylenol) is a very safe medication when given in normal doses to infants and children, and it has few adverse effects. However, if too much acetaminophen is given—if a toxic dose is given—acetaminophen can cause liver failure and be fatal.

It is also important to evaluate "benefit-to-risk" considerations for your child's medicines. As with nearly everything in life, there are benefits and risks in what we do. The benefits, which should be greater than the risks, include things like reducing a fever, curing an infection, improving breathing difficulties from asthma, or preventing a seizure. The risks entail medication adverse effects, which often are not serious or are manageable. However, some *can* be serious. When the benefits to children of some medications or supplements are not proven, then the risks are greater than the benefits. Examples include OTC antidiarrheal medicines and many supplements (see chapter 3 for more information). *This is a very important concept to understand and appreciate.* Studies of pediatric medication adverse effects are described later in this chapter.

As Needed, or Every Day?

An important distinction to know about your child's medicine is whether it should be given on a regular daily schedule or only as needed. Medicines for fever, such as acetaminophen (Tylenol) and ibuprofen (Motrin, Advil), are typically given as needed, when your child is uncomfortable or has a high body temperature. Other medicines should *not* be given only as needed, and are most effective when given daily, even if the child feels well and has no apparent symptoms from the illness. Examples of medications scheduled for every day administration are many asthma medicines, such as Flovent (fluticasone) or Singulair (montelukast), and many medicines for seizure disorders, such as Tegretol (carbamazepine) or Dilantin (phenytoin). It is easy to confuse some asthma medicines, such as some metered dose inhalers (Proair [albuterol] or Proventil [albuterol]), which are mostly given as needed when the child has difficulty breathing. Other metered dose inhalers, such as Flovent (fluticasone), should be used every day, whether or not the child has breathing difficulty, and are not effective when used only as needed.

The Art of Giving Medicine to Children

All parents know the difficulties of giving medicine to infants and children. Beyond these relatively "simple" difficulties are potential problems that many parents may not be aware of, such as accurately measuring liquid doses. Most medicines given to infants and young children are liquids. Accurately measuring a dose of these liquid medicines is important and, as studies have shown, it can be quite difficult. Beyond accurately measuring a dose of liquid medicine comes the "art" of getting your infant or young child to take the medicine. Color, texture, smell, and, perhaps most important, taste of the liquid medicine all come into play. What can be done to entice your child to take his or her medicine?

Dosing Devices

I recall my mother giving me liquid medicine on a teaspoon when I was a young child. We have known for many years that this is not an accurate way to measure and give medicine. The pediatric medical community and professional medical organizations have recently published specific recommendations stating not to use kitchen teaspoons or tablespoons to give liquid medicine. Back in 1975 the Committee on Drugs of the American Academy of Pediatrics (AAP) stated in a report titled "Inaccuracies of Administering Liquid Medication" that "teaspoons are particularly poor measuring and administering devices." This report also discussed how much the size of kitchen teaspoons varies, delivering between 50 percent and 156 percent of the amount medically considered to be a teaspoonful, which is 5 mL (milliliters). Other studies have found that teaspoons vary in their delivery of liquids by 60 percent to 180 percent.

In 2015, 40 years later, the AAP Committee on Drugs published a similar report again advising that kitchen or household teaspoons and tablespoons not be used to measure and deliver liquid medicines. This report also recommended that pediatricians and other prescribers stop writing prescriptions using teaspoon or tablespoon amounts. Unfortunately, some prescribers continue to write prescriptions this way. Several studies have documented that, when given the opportunity to choose a dosing device to measure liquid medicine, many parents choose a household teaspoon instead of other, more accurate, dosing devices. The 2015 AAP report included several important recommendations:

- Oral liquid medicine volumes should be expressed with metric system units, such as mL (milliliters), not with teaspoonsful or tablespoonsful.
- Pharmacy bottle labels should state volumes as mL and not teaspoon or tablespoon, for example, "Give 5 mL twice a day," not "Give 1 teaspoonful twice a day."
- Accurate dosing devices should be given to parents with all liquid medicines.

What are accurate measuring devices? Dosing devices evaluated in published studies include oral syringes, cylindrical spoons, droppers, and dosing cups. Several studies have demonstrated oral syringes to be the most accurate. Dosing cups, which are typically made of plastic and available with OTC liquid medication product packages, are often kept in homes and re-used by parents for giving different liquid medicines to their children. When comparing the accuracy of measuring 5 mL liquid volumes with dosing cups and oral syringes by parents, a study in 2008 and another in 2016 found dosing errors to be four times and five times more likely when dosing cups were used, as compared to when oral syringes were used. One of these studies also demonstrated that even though oral syringes were more accurate, only 67 percent of parents using them correctly measured an accurate dose, indicating that even oral syringes can be frequently used improperly or inaccurately.

Explanations of dosing technique given by parents enrolled in these studies is revealing. Some parents confused "teaspoonful" with "tablespoonful" (a tablespoonful is 15 mL, three times greater than a teaspoonful, 5 mL), and others believed a full dosing cup was the standard dose. In summary, practical recommendations from these studies include the following suggestions:

- Request an oral dosing syringe at the pharmacy for your child's liquid medicine, and ask to be shown where on the syringe to measure your child's dose (one published study demonstrated this as the most accurate method).
- Consider a smaller size oral syringe if you are administering liquid medicine to an infant. Smaller syringes are more accurate when measuring smaller liquid doses. Oral syringes can be especially useful when administering liquid medicine to your infant, as you can place the syringe just inside your infant's mouth and he or she will naturally begin sucking the medicine out.
- Consider other dosing devices sold in pharmacies—droppers and dosing spoons, although they may not be as accurate or as easy to use as an oral syringe.

- Avoid using dosing cups, since they are not as accurate as measuring devices and it's best not to use them to measure most liquid medicines; exceptions can include larger volumes of liquid for older children or adolescents.
- Use mL (milliliters) for measuring liquid medicines, not teaspoonsful or tablespoonsful, and ask your pediatrician and pharmacist to clarify your child's medicine dose as mL.
- Take extra care when measuring and administering liquid medications. Studies of parents have shown it can be easy to make errors when giving liquid medicine to children.

Taste of Liquid Medicines

The taste of liquid medicine is an important factor when administering medications to children. An effective medicine will not help your child if he or she refuses to take it, which can be frustrating. Pharmaceutical manufacturers strive to make their liquid medicine products appealing to children, focusing not just on taste but also considering the appearance or color, smell, texture, and viscosity. Fortunately, most liquid medicines given to children taste relatively good. Some medicines, however, are chemically bitter and this is hard to mask in a liquid medicine product. Several taste tests of liquid medicine products have been published, mostly focusing on antibiotics. Antibiotics that adults rated as tasting good in these taste tests include:

- amoxicillin
- amoxicillin-clavulanate acid (Augmentin)
- cefdinir (Omnicef)
- cefprozil (Cefzil)
- azithromycin (Zithromax)

Medications scoring less well on taste (that is, testers did *not* like their taste) include:

- cefpodoxime (Vantin)

- cefuroxime (Ceftin)
- clarithromycin (Biaxin)
- penicillin
- clindamycin
- some prednisolone products (the product Orapred may taste better)

What can you do if your child's pediatrician prescribes one of the medications above that does not taste good? Several methods may help your child successfully take the medicine. The following tips may be helpful:

- Ask your pharmacist to flavor the medicine.

Many pharmacies have standardized flavoring systems, such as FlavorRx, that utilize many different flavors to add to a liquid medication. They may charge an additional fee for this (usually about $3 extra). FlavorRx offers a variety of flavorings for liquid medication products that may be appealing to your child, such as chocolate, mango, orange, and watermelon. Your child can choose from bubblegum, grape, raspberry, or grape-bubblegum flavor enhancers to improve the taste of Vantin (cefpodoxime), an antibiotic commonly prescribed for children with ear infections. Ask if your pharmacy is able to do this.

- Offer your child a teaspoonful of sweet syrup before or after administering the medicine.

Try giving your child a teaspoonful of chocolate (or butterscotch, strawberry, or maple) syrup just before and after giving the liquid medicine. This may help "bribe" your child, as it tastes good, and the syrup can coat the tongue and help to mask the liquid medicine taste. You can also try honey, as it has a sweet flavor. A word of caution, though—do not give honey to infants younger than 1 year of age, as it may contain certain bacterial spores that can be dangerous to young infants. Some strong-tasting juices, such as grape juice (purple or white), can be similarly used, to give before and after the liquid medicine, to help mask its taste.

• Mix the liquid with applesauce, pudding, or jellies/jams.

If you try mixing a liquid with applesauce, pudding, or jellies, be sure to mix them well together. In addition, be careful not to use too much, as your child may not want to finish all of it, and consequently won't get the full dose of medicine. Use enough, however, to mask the medicine taste.

• Give a popsicle or refrigerate the medicine.

Many liquids, such as orange juice, taste best when cold, and chilling your child's medicine can also help it taste better. Ask your pharmacist if your child's liquid medicine can be refrigerated. It is important to ask, because some liquid antibiotics, such as clarithromycin (Biaxin), should *not* be refrigerated (it can thicken up a lot when stored in a refrigerator). Giving a popsicle before the medicine can also be helpful, as a cold tongue may not detect the liquid medicine taste as much.

• Give a good tasting liquid or nutritional formula just after the medicine.

Give another liquid that your child likes, such as milk or juice, or your infant's nutritional formula, just after the liquid medicine, as this can help flush the medicine taste out of the mouth.

• Give your child's liquid medicine when he or she is likely to be hungry.

Your child is more likely to eat and drink when he or she is hungry. Check with your pharmacist to be sure that the medicine can be given with food or the drinks discussed above, as some medicines are best absorbed on an empty stomach (1 hour before or 2 hours after a meal).

- Try mixing your child's medicine in with nutritional formula or expressed breast milk (in the same bottle) or in with a liquid that your child likes, such as chocolate milk.

Check with your pharmacist first to be sure that there are no problems with mixing the medicine this way (you want to avoid affecting the medication's chemical stability). Don't use too much formula or liquid since your child may not finish the full amount and consequently will not get all of the liquid medicine. For example, if your infant normally has 6 to 8 ounces of formula per feeding, try mixing about 3 ounces of formula with the medicine (when he or she is likely to be hungry), and then give the remaining amount of formula.

- Invest in a novel delivery device.

If you're still having trouble getting your child to take the medicine, you can try some interesting and helpful devices available online (and perhaps in your pharmacy) that function by giving liquid medicines together with nutritional formula or other liquids, such as pumped breast milk. Some of these devices combine an oral dosing syringe within a bottle and nipple, so the formula or milk is taken together with the liquid medicine. Examples include Medibottle, Reliadose, and Munchkin. Another device, Pacidose, combines a pacifier directly with an oral dosing syringe, to encourage an infant or young child to take the liquid medicine. These devices seem reasonable to try.

This discussion of liquid medicine taste has centered on prescription liquid medicines. Your child may also not like the taste of some liquid OTC products, such as acetaminophen (Tylenol) or ibuprofen (Motrin, Advil). Similar to some prescription medications, OTC medication products are available as trade products, such as Tylenol, and as generic products. Many retail pharmacy chains or pharmacies located in grocery store chains carry their own generic brand. Either the trade or generic product can be used, although generic products are likely to be less expensive. Their taste, however, may differ from the trade products, similar to trade and generic prescription medication products. I recall when my son was young and had a fever. We were out of Tylenol, so I went to the pharmacy to buy more (of course it was late at night). I noticed that a generic form of infant's acetaminophen was much less expensive than the trade product, Tylenol, and I bought several boxes of the generic product. Well, my son must not have liked the taste because he wouldn't take the generic product. Back to the pharmacy I went to buy the trade product Tylenol. He liked this better and took it easily. I tried the tastes of both, and I agreed that the trade product, Tylenol, tasted better than the generic product.

When giving an OTC liquid product to your child, use the dosing device that comes with the package, as this device should match the product package dosing instructions and you will be less likely to make an error when measuring an appropriate dose for your child's weight.

Techniques for Giving Liquid Medicine

Technique makes a difference when giving any liquid medicine. Use an oral dosing syringe and slowly administer the liquid toward the side of your child's mouth, not directly on the tongue (where the taste buds are). In this way the medicine flows toward your child's throat, is more easily swallowed, and bypasses the taste buds. Do not quickly squirt the liquid medicine into the back of your child's mouth, as he or she may choke. Young children may want to help by holding the oral syringe or by sucking the medicine out of the syringe. If for some reason your child does not seem to be swallowing the medicine, you can try gently holding his or her cheeks together and then lightly stroking under the chin. When administering liquid medicine to infants, have another adult hold the infant, including his or her arms. Older infants or young children can be placed in an infant car seat or high chair used for eating. When you are done, rinse the oral syringe with water. Don't let your child play with the dosing syringe, as he or she could potentially choke on it. Store it in a safe place.

Giving Tablets and Capsules to Your Child

A common question parents ask is, "When should my child be able to swallow a tablet or capsule?" There is no specific age when a child *should* be able to swallow a tablet or capsule. I've seen some 2-year-olds who can swallow tablets, and some adolescents who can't. Several pediatric medicine textbooks state that by age 6 or 7 years, most children are able to swallow tablets, but this varies widely and is not a golden rule.

If your child is unable to swallow a tablet whole, don't fret. There are several options you may try. Perhaps the easiest is to cut the tablet into two halves or even four quarters and let your child try swallowing these smaller pieces. Many medicine tablets are "scored"— they have a line in the middle of the tablet that can be used to more easily break the tablet into two pieces. You may be able to do this with your fingers, or you could use a tablet splitter (available at most pharmacies for a few dollars). Some tablet medications should *not* be broken or split (for example, coated tablets or slow-release tablets), so check with your pharmacist before doing this. You may ask your pharmacy to split all of your child's tablets when you first pick up the prescription, or call in a refill. Some pharmacies will gladly do this, while others will not, but it is reasonable to ask.

Some medications, such as amoxicillin and amoxicillin-clavulanate (Augmentin), are also available as chewable tablets or tablets that dissolve quickly in the mouth, and they typically taste good. Another option is to crush the tablet into many small pieces or a powder and give this. While this is commonly recommended, it can be hard to do and may not be accurate, since it can be difficult to gather up the entire crushed tablet pieces. If you try this, it is best to crush the tablet in a small bowl (or use a tablet crushing device sold in pharmacies) and then mix the small pieces together well with jelly or jam and give this to your child. When you mix medicines with food as described here and above with liquid medicines, always give the mixture to your child immediately after you prepare it, and do not save it for later or prepare doses ahead of time. Because of potential chemical instability, mixing medicines like this several hours in advance may affect the potency of the medication. In addition, check with your pharmacist to be sure that your child's medicine can be given with food and is not supposed to be taken on an empty stomach.

Some medicine products are also available as capsules that can be easily opened up and sprinkled onto food and given this way. Your child's pediatrician is likely familiar with these pediatric sprinkle capsule dosage forms, but you can ask if your child's medicine is available as a sprinkle capsule. The type of food that many of these sprinkle capsule dosage forms are given with is important, so be sure to ask about this at the pharmacy. Most capsules are not specifically designed to be sprinkled onto food, although the contents of some capsules can be mixed with food. The powder contents are likely to taste bitter or bad, however, so mix it with a food that has a strong good taste, such as jelly or jam. Check with your pharmacist before doing this, to make sure there are no chemical stability problems.

If you want to help your older child swallow his or her tablets or capsules, several devices may be useful. A review of this subject published in 2014 found that certain head posture techniques, behavioral therapies, flavored throat sprays, and swallow tablet cups were effective. The head posture techniques and behavioral techniques are too complex to fully explain here, and are likely best demonstrated by and practiced with supervision by health care professionals at children's hospitals located in large cities. A device that can help children (and adults) swallow tablets and capsules is Oralflo. This device looks like a children's sippy cup and has a pocket inside to place the tablet or capsule. When the cup is filled with liquid, the medicine more easily slides out with the liquid, to be swallowed. Another aid that can be tried is Pill Glide, a lubricant sprayed into the mouth that reduces friction between the medicine and throat and mouth, helping the tablet or capsule slide and be swallowed more easily.

Other Issues When Giving Medicine to Children
Your Child Vomits After Taking Medicine

Once your child has swallowed his or her medicine, thanks in large part to your efforts in preparing the medicine and coaxing him or her, it's always possible that soon after, he or she will vomit. What do you do then? Should you give another dose, or out of fear of giving too much medicine, let it be? This depends on several factors, including the specific medicine given and the time between giving the medicine and your child vomiting. Parents are often told if it has been less than 1 hour since giving a medication, another dose can be administered. This may not apply to all medicines, however. Liquid medicines are absorbed into the bloodstream faster than tablets or capsules. Most liquid medicines are absorbed in less than 1 hour, and if your child vomits 45 minutes after swallowing a liquid medicine, another dose is likely not necessary.

If the medication was a tablet, it can be helpful to look at your child's vomit for visible pieces of the tablet. If you see some, much of the tablet probably was not absorbed. It is also important to consider the specific medication your child was given, and its potential for adverse effects. Some medications can cause significantly more adverse effects with only one or two doses above the current dose, while other medications, such as many antibiotics, are unlikely to cause more adverse effects with one or two extra doses. Check with your pediatrician before giving more medicine after your child has vomited.

Giving Medicine with or without Food

Some medications are best given on an empty stomach, as food in the stomach delays or reduces how much of the medication is absorbed into the blood. An example is penicillin, the antibiotic of choice for strep throat infections. Penicillin is best absorbed with an empty stomach, although it can be given with food, if nausea occurs. Another antibiotic best given without food is tetracycline. Because dairy products bind with tetracycline in the stomach and reduce how much is absorbed, they should be especially avoided. Infants and children seem to be hungry nearly all of the time, and they can have food in their stomachs most hours of the day. If a medicine should be given on an empty stomach, which is typically described as 1 hour before a meal or 2 hours after a meal, the timing of giving the medicine with your child's eating can be quite difficult.

Other medications are best given *with* food, as food increases the amount of medication absorbed, or more commonly, food reduces the likelihood of nausea or vomiting occurring. Amoxicillin-clavu-lanate (Augmentin), an antibiotic commonly used in pediatrics, is best given with food to decrease the potential for adverse effects of nausea, vomiting, or diarrhea. The antifungal medication griseofulvin is best given with food, since food increases the amount absorbed.

Whether to give some medicines with or without food can also depend on the dosage form of the medicine, and not the medicine per se. Fortunately, whether to give a medication with or without food is not significantly important for many medicines. Your pharmacy will counsel you on how your child's medicine is best given, with or without food, or either. If you are not sure, ask your pharmacist.

Giving Medicine at School or Daycare

Your child may need someone at school or daycare to administer his or her medicine. Schools and daycare establishments have widely varying policies about giving medicine to children, and it is best to contact your child's school or daycare before you send medicine along with him or her. Your child's school or daycare medicine should be sent in a regular pharmacy-labeled container, similar to what the pharmacy normally dispenses. Ask the pharmacy to place your child's medicine into similar home and school or daycare bottles and vials with labels. The pharmacy will place various stickers on the vials as necessary, such as "Take with Food," or "Store in the Refrigerator," which will help ensure that the medicine is given properly.

Do not send your child to school with medicine in a baggie or other nonpharmacy containers, even if the medicine is an OTC medication such as ibuprofen (Motrin, Advil). Nursing offices at schools have bottles of these common OTC medications when a child is in need, such as for headache or other mild pain. The school nurse will likely call you for approval before giving any medicine, or you may be asked in advance to sign an authorization form.

All schools should allow your child to carry his or her asthma inhaler (such as albuterol), to be used as needed when your child has breathing difficulties. Your child may need access to this inhaler quickly when breathing difficulties begin. The school will probably require a signed consent note from you and your pediatrician allowing this use, and the school nurse may ask your child to demonstrate that he or she can properly use the inhaler. Inhalers are best sent properly labeled with a pharmacy label attached directly on the inhaler, and not just on the inhaler product box. Schools may also allow other medicines to be carried by a child, if this medicine is necessary for quick use by the child for a specific medical condition. Speak with your child's pediatrician and school to determine this.

States have varying policies for allowing medicine to be given at daycare establishments. If your infant or young child attends daycare, speak with the daycare personnel before sending medicine. Just as in a school setting, you will need to sign a consent allowing the medicine to be given, and the medicine should be correctly labeled. The daycare workers should be properly trained to administer medicines. Ask about this. Your local or state health department can be a valuable information source about your state's laws regulating daycare establishments.

Adherence: The Importance of Taking Medicine

There are numerous reasons why children do not receive all of the medicine that is prescribed for them, including forgetting, concerns about adverse effects, cost of the medicine, belief that the medicine is no longer necessary once the child has begun to feel better, misunderstanding the directions, or a stigma associated with taking some medicines (such as antidepressants), among others. Forgetting doses is perhaps the most common reason, and it easily occurs, especially in a busy home or lifestyle. *Nonadherence* is the term used to describe not taking medicines as prescribed or recommended. Recognizing the potential for nonadherence with your child's medicines is very important, and some relatively simple solutions can help you avoid many of the causes of reduced adherence.

The majority of children—63 percent—diagnosed with a chronic illness are prescribed at least one medicine. Unfortunately, studies have demonstrated that 50 to 88 percent of children who have a chronic illness, such as asthma or diabetes, do not take all of their prescribed medicine. Even though common sense suggests this, many studies have documented that medication adherence for asthma and diabetes, and other serious conditions, is beneficial, since children taking their medicine are less likely to be admitted to a hospital and are healthier. Numerous studies have been published in the medical literature about adherence to medication and other illness treatment recommendations given by physicians and health care professionals. Overall, these studies suggest that beneficial strategies can be used by parents to improve medication adherence and their child's health. Strategies that parents can employ are described as behavioral and educational.

Behavioral strategies include instituting reminders to prevent missed doses because of forgetfulness, such as setting phone alarms, using pill boxes, or posting notes in your home. I frequently suggest to parents and adolescent patients that they link taking their medicine with a personal habit that is already established, such as teeth brushing. Place the medication vial next to your child's toothbrush, as a visual reminder. Rewarding your young child when medicine is taken can also be helpful. Children and adolescents with a chronic disease such as asthma or diabetes can significantly benefit from involvement in local or national organizations representing the illness, as these organizations often have peer and parent support groups with local meetings where participants can hear from other parents about their success stories or frustrations with giving medicine to their children.

Educational strategies can also be helpful. These include being sure that you completely understand how your child's medicine is appropriately given, including the information listed in table 2.1. This may seem rather simplistic, but it is important. I have spoken with many parents or adolescents who misunderstood how their medicine was supposed to be taken, and they mistakenly took the medicine only once daily instead of twice daily, as prescribed. It is easy to get confused, especially when you are given a lot of information in the pediatrician's office and in the pharmacy when the medicine is initially prescribed. A common problem I hear from parents relates to missing doses. Nearly everyone likely misses occasional doses of his or her medicine, but if it happens frequently, the doses missed can significantly add up and decrease the medicine's benefit. Be sure to ask your pharmacist and pediatrician what you should do if you miss a dose of your child's medicine. For many medications, the missed dose can safely be given later.

Studies have shown the simpler the medication directions or regimen, the better—that is, the more likely that the medicine will be given. For example, adherence to a medicine that is dosed three times daily is likely to be less than to a medicine that is dosed twice daily. Discuss dosing schedules with your pediatrician, and ask your pharmacist how you can adapt your child's medicine regimen to your daily home lifestyle. These discussions can be very helpful to you. Nonadherence with medication reaches a peak in the adolescent years—a time that can be very frustrating to parents. Being aware of this potential, and discussing it with your adolescent's pediatrician, can be helpful.

It is important to be honest with your pediatrician and pharmacist when they ask about medication adherence. No one likes to be thought of as a "bad parent," but if your child is not receiving all of his or her medicine, your doctor needs to know. Health care professionals understand the difficulties of giving medicines to children or adolescents. Sharing your difficulties and concerns about your child's medicine will likely be very helpful, as your pharmacist and pediatrician will be able to suggest methods for improvement. I have heard from parents and adolescents about their concerns with a medicine's adverse effects, and at times they have been reluctant to admit that their source was what they read on the Internet or what a neighbor may have told them about their child's medicine (which often is misleading or false). Occasionally, cost and paying for medicines may be a concern, especially as medicine costs are rising and health insurance drug coverage is decreasing. If cost is a concern, pediatricians and pharmacists may well be able to help, by prescribing less expensive medicines or by utilizing pharmaceutical company rebates and discounts.

Benefits versus Risks of Medicine

As discussed previously in this chapter, giving any medicine to your child involves certain benefits and risks. Benefits of giving medicine include helping your child feel better (reducing pain or fever), treating a chronic illness (such as asthma), or curing an infection (such as an ear infection). These benefits can be large and potentially life-saving. Risks and disadvantages of giving medicine involve medication adverse effects, allergic reactions, a potential for toxicity or poisoning, difficulties of giving the medicine, and cost, among others. The benefits should be greater than the risks; otherwise, the medicine is best not given.

In this section, I explore this principle more closely, and discuss the many studies that have evaluated medication adverse effects and other risks in large populations of children. One of the main points that this discussion will lead to is this: *all* medicines have a potential for risk. It is common in our society to treat nearly any symptom or any illness we have, even minor illnesses, with medicine. Children are not small adults, and the risks of using medicine in children can be greater than the benefits for some illnesses (these will be explained in more detail throughout this book). Thus, if a medication is unlikely to help your child, and as it may cause adverse effects or other risks, it is best not used. This is an important principle.

Several recently published studies have evaluated and documented medication risks in pediatrics. A study published in 2014 analyzed medication errors that occurred in settings outside of a hospital (at home or other areas) in children over an 11-year period. During this time, 696,937 children younger than 6 years of age experienced a medication error—this averaged to a medication error occurring every 8 minutes! The errors included accidentally giving a medicine twice and giving incorrect doses or measuring doses inaccurately, among others. In this study, the younger the child, the greater the likelihood of a medication error occurring—25 percent of all the errors occurred in infants younger than 1 year of age, and 25 children died as a result of these errors.

In a study published in 2008 the researchers evaluated visits to hospital emergency departments because of adverse effects from antibiotic use in children and adults over a 3-year period. The majority, 79 percent, of the 6,614 cases identified were due to allergic reactions from the antibiotic. Children 14 years of age and younger accounted for 25 percent of all of the cases. The highest rate of antibiotic allergic reactions occurred in infants younger than 12 months of age. When these occurrence rates are extrapolated to all hospitals in the United States, 37,000 visits by children 14 years of age and younger to hospital emergency departments occur each year because of adverse effects from antibiotic use.

In an article published in 2013, the authors reviewed 11 published studies about medication-related emergency department visits and hospital admissions (described as adverse medication events in this study) in the pediatric population. The researchers found that adverse reactions, overdoses, and allergic reactions were the most common occurrences, with antibiotics the most common class of medication responsible. Perhaps most important, the researchers determined that 20 to 67 percent of the adverse medication events were preventable. Many additional published studies have shown that the most common medication error that occurs in infants and children involves errors with medication dosing.

What do these studies tell us? They reveal that medicine use in children, and especially in infants and younger children, can result in many unwanted and potentially serious—including death—adverse effects. It is best not to give medicine to your infant or child unless it will benefit them. Discuss benefits and risks with your pediatrician and pharmacist before a new medicine is begun and given to your child. Ask what the benefits and risks of the medicine are, and if the benefits will be greater than the risks. Ask what safer nonmedication treatments you may be able to use to help your child feel better.

Protecting Your Child from Medicine Poisonings

Because young children are curious, active, and mobile (and have a tendency to put nearly anything in their mouths) they are at higher risk from accidental poisonings. More than 500,000 children 5 years of age and younger experience a poisoning exposure each year. This risk peaks at about age 2 years of age. There are many relatively simple changes you can make in your home, where most poisonings occur, to reduce the risk of your child experiencing an accidental poisoning. Several good Internet sites, including www.poisonprevention.org and www.healthychildren.org, list specific details of how to poison proof a home.

Medicines are a leading cause of accidental poisonings. Most homes contain several medicines that can be fatal to a young child if enough medicine is swallowed, including acetaminophen (Tylenol), aspirin, and iron (including vitamins containing iron). Many prescription medications commonly used by adults can be especially dangerous, including some antidepressants (such as amitriptyline), medications for heart problems and pain, and medications for high blood sugar. Just 1 or 2 tablets of some of these medications can be fatal to a 2-year-old child.

While young adult parents may not use these medications, they may be taken by grandparents and other older adults who frequently spend time with the children. A scenario that can easily occur involves young children visiting their grandparents, and while the adults congregate in the kitchen or family room, the young children somehow manage to find grandma's or grandpa's medicine bottles (more than 50 percent of grandparents have easy-open tops on their medicine bottles) and swallow several tablets. Other medicines that many may not consider dangerous include methyl salicylate and camphor. Methyl salicylate can be applied to skin (one example is Bengay) to reduce pain or it can be used as a food-flavoring agent, as oil of wintergreen. Camphor is an active ingredient in Vicks Vapo Rub (for treatment of cough in children) and if swallowed, just 20 mL (about 1 tablespoonful) can be fatal to a 2-year-old child. Less than 5 mL (less than 1 teaspoonful) of concentrated oil of wintergreen can be fatal to a 2-year-old child.

Pediatricians commonly include a discussion on home poison proofing with parents when infants are about 6 months of age, as they then begin to become more mobile by crawling. The information shared with you by your pediatrician and information from the Internet sites listed above can be very helpful, and it may potentially save your child's life. It's also important to know the national poison control center phone number—800-222-1222—and keep it in a handy place. By calling this phone number, you will be directed to your local poison control center, regardless of where you live in the United States. If your child is exposed to a potential poison, call this phone number before calling your pediatrician, as poison control centers employ health care professionals specifically trained in the treatment of poisonings. If your child is not breathing or is unconscious, call 911.

Generic Medicines: Are They Safe and Effective?

The short answer to this question is, yes. Generic medicines are equally safe and effective as the equivalent brand name medicine and are usually significantly less expensive than the brand name medicine. Generic medicines must be demonstrated to be bioequivalent to the same brand name medication (the amount of medication absorbed and distributed to the medication's site of action) and to be as safe as the brand name medication. The FDA regulates generic medicines similarly to brand name medicines. The FDA ensures that generic medications have the same active ingredients, strength, purity, and quality as the brand name product.

About 80 percent of all prescriptions in the United States are generic medicines, and most generic medicines cost 80 to 85 percent less than the brand name medicine. When a brand name medication loses its patent or exclusivity (exclusive rights to market a medication product by a pharmaceutical manufacturer), the cost of the first available generic medication is usually not significantly lower. The medication's price decreases only about 6 months later, when other generic companies begin producing additional generic versions of the medication. Most generic versions of a medication will appear different in color, size, or shape than the brand name product. However, when the same pharmaceutical manufacturer produces a generic version of its own brand product, to sell at a lower price, the generic medication may look very similar to the brand product.

All states allow generic medications to be dispensed, although these laws may differ among states. The FDA publishes a standardized book (the "Orange Book") that pharmacies use to determine which generic medications are bioequivalent to brand name medications. I often hear parents express concerns that a generic medication is not the same, or will not work the same, as the brand name medication. While I certainly understand their concerns, I tell them that the generic medication should treat their child's condition just as effectively and safely as the brand name product, as both are well regulated by the FDA for purity and content.

Some medications have a narrow therapeutic index, which implies that the difference between the medication's efficacy and toxicity are narrower than most medications. When a medication with a narrow therapeutic index is used, either a blood level of the medication or another parameter in the blood is carefully measured and monitored to ensure that the medication concentration in the blood does not increase to a toxic amount. If a child is receiving a medication with a narrow therapeutic index and is doing well, it may not be wise to change from the manufacturer of this medication to a different generic or brand name manufacturer. Your pediatrician and pharmacist will discuss this with you. Examples of these medicines include some that treat seizure disorders, such as Dilantin (phenytoin) or Tegretol (carbamazepine).

If a medication prescribed for your child is expensive, ask your pediatrician and pharmacist if a generic version is available. If not, ask your pediatrician if a medication is available generically that will be just as effective and safe as the prescribed medication. The answer is often yes. For example, an older medicine in the same medication class may be just as effective as the new, more expensive medication.

The Rising Cost of Medicines

The rising cost of medicine became a top news story in 2015, and it continues to be a headline on televised national news programs and in newspapers. How pharmaceutical manufacturers determine medication prices is quite complex. As with other commodities that we consume, a lack of competition for specific medications drives prices up, since a pharmaceutical manufacturer can charge exorbitant prices when it is the only supplier of a product. This has occurred with several medicines recently, resulting in price increases of up to 6,000 percent when competition for a medicine dwindles.

Many factors determine what you pay at the pharmacy, including competition (multiple pharmaceutical manufacturers producing the same medication), health insurance coverage (copay and deductible amounts), and availability of a generic form, among others. When a medication is available in more than one generic form, it is likely to be significantly less expensive. When a new medication is manufactured and is not available generically, it is likely to be expensive. All medications can be placed into categories or medication classes, according to what they are used to treat (this is called their "indication") and their pharmacology (their mechanism of action or how they function). When new medications are introduced, quite often older medications within the same class that function similarly continue to be available and are often less expensive. New medications are not always better, and their high prices may not be justified. Medications within the same class can differ to some extent, such as one may be given once daily, as compared to others in the same class given twice or three times daily. This can be an important characteristic, and may justify a medication's higher cost.

Insurance companies often dictate to a large extent what price you will pay at the pharmacy. For example, an insurance company may decide not to pay for a new, expensive medication when it is prescribed for its insured members. If your child were prescribed this medication by your pediatrician, you would be charged a high price for it. The insurance company would likely pay for similar, less expensive, medicines within the same medication class, and thus your price at the pharmacy would be lower. Insurance companies maintain drug formularies, a listing of prescription drugs within a class or category, including the amount of the drug cost they will cover, and how much you will pay. Your pediatrician may be able to prescribe a medication for your child that is preferred by the insurance company, saving you money.

What can you do to avoid paying higher costs for your child's medicines? When a medication is prescribed for your child, discuss the cost of the medication with your pediatrician. If it is expensive, ask if a less expensive medication can be used that will be just as likely to help your child. Ask if a generic form of the medication is available and can be prescribed. Your pediatrician's office staff may be able to check your insurance company's Internet site for specific medications covered under your plan, or you can call your insurance company and ask for this information. Many OTC medications are also available as generic, less expensive, products. Ask your pharmacist to help you choose one that is best for your child. Many patient assistance programs are available that you may qualify for, allowing you to save money on prescription drug costs. These programs can be viewed on several Internet sites:

- Partnership for Prescription Assistance, www.pparx.org
  ◊ access to more than 475 public and private patient assistance programs
- RxAssist, www.rxassist.org
  ◊ listing of numerous patient assistance programs
- NeedyMeds, www.needymeds.org
  ◊ listing of numerous patient assistance programs

Expired Medications

It is best not to use an expired medicine. However, the convenience of choosing to use a medication in your home which has a recent expiration date (say, several months ago) versus driving to a pharmacy late at night or in bad weather is also important to consider. In many circumstances, using the expired medicine until you are able to buy new medicine is likely a reasonable and safe option.

The pharmaceutical manufacturer's expiration date is usually stamped in print on the bottom or side of the bottle or box for OTC medications, and may appear as something like *EXP 10/16*. Products that contain medications that are applied to the skin, such as lotions or skin protectants may not have an expiration date on the box or product. For prescription medications obtained at your pharmacy, the expiration date will likely be one year from the date it is dispensed, even when the original product bottle the pharmacy used had an expiration date of more than one year. A one-year expiration date will be placed on your bottle because how you store the medicine cannot be guaranteed to be appropriate. Storage conditions, such as temperature, humidity, and light, can greatly affect a product's expiration date. The most appropriate conditions to store most medicines are a cool, dry place, with low humidity. Unfortunately, most medicines are likely stored in our bathrooms—not a good place because of the high humidity. A better place to store many medicines is in a clothing drawer, where it is cool, dry, and dark.

Use of a medication with an expiration date long since passed may result in the medicine not functioning as well, due to loss of strength or potency. Consumers may be concerned that an expired medication may somehow morph or change into a toxic or dangerous substance, but this is unfounded.

Several published studies have evaluated medication expiration dates and tested medication potency at times significantly longer than the product's expiration date. These studies found that when stored in the medication's original, sealed container at room temperature, many medications retain their original potency for many years beyond the manufacturer's labeled expiration dates. However, it is also important to consider that nearly all medications given to your child are not in their original container and are not stored under ideal conditions. How you store medicine—away from humidity, light, and high or low temperatures, and with the vial or bottle top tightly in place—can significantly affect the expiration time and potency of the medicine.

The intended use of a medication is an additional important consideration. Medications that may greatly affect your child's health with each dose, such as insulin or epinephrine auto injectors for severe allergies, should not be used past their indicated expiration date, even when they are stored under good conditions. If your child uses one of these medications, or a medication for a similar purpose, it is best to be aware of the medication's expiration date and obtain a refill at the pharmacy or a new prescription from your pediatrician well ahead of the expiration date. It may be reasonable and safe to use other medication products, such as acetaminophen (Tylenol) or ibuprofen (Motrin, Advil), with recent past expiration dates, when giving one or two doses is not as critical to your child's health, and when you are realistically unable to obtain more medicine immediately.

Summary Points for Parents

- Dosing errors are the most common drug error in pediatrics. Determine an accurate dose for all OTC drugs given to your infant or child. Ask your pharmacist to help you if need be.

- Use an accurate dosing device to measure your child's liquid medicine. Do not use teaspoons or tablespoons. As many parents easily make mistakes measuring liquid medicine, don't hesitate to ask your pharmacist to show you how best to measure your child's dose.

- Your child may not like the taste of a liquid medicine and may refuse to take it. Your pharmacy may be able to flavor your child's medicine and improve the taste.

- Before giving any new prescription or OTC drug to your child, consider if, and how, the drug will help your child, and what adverse effects it may cause. All drugs have potential to result in adverse effects, and some may be severe. The benefit of any drug given to your child should be greater than the adverse effects.

- It can be easy to make mistakes when giving medicine to your child, such as missing doses. Discuss how to appropriately give a new medicine to your child with your pediatrician and pharmacist, and know what questions to ask.

- Some medicines can be very expensive. Less expensive medicines are often just as likely to help your child. Know what questions to ask your pediatrician and pharmacist about the cost of your child's medicine.

3

Over-the-Counter, Herbal, Supplement, and Vitamin Products

In this chapter, I provide information that you should have about over-the-counter (OTC), herbal, alternative, and vitamin products before giving them to your children. Although OTC drug products are generally regarded as safe to use without a physician's approval or prescription, they continue to have potential for serious adverse effects or toxicity if not given correctly. Herbal and alternative products, which are not well regulated and are heavily marketed, may not produce the benefits for your child that manufacturers would like you to believe.

Parents often give OTC medicines to infants and children, most commonly acetaminophen (Tylenol) or ibuprofen (Motrin, Advil) to treat fever. Because OTC medicines are, by definition, available without a prescription, it is not necessary to speak with a pharmacist or pediatrician before administering them. Getting advice from your pharmacist or pediatrician would certainly be helpful, however, because administration of OTC medicines can result in adverse effects, some potentially serious. Published studies have shown that parents easily make mistakes when giving OTC products to their children. Some OTC medicines, although marketed and available as pediatric products, are best not given to children.

The use of herbal products, alternative medicines, and vitamin products in adults and children has increased in recent years. Unlike prescription and OTC medicines, herbal and vitamin products and alternative medicines are not stringently regulated by the Food and Drug Administration (FDA). This lack of regulation has significant implications for their potential safe use and raises questions about their effectiveness.

Over-the-Counter Medical Products
Regulation

OTC medicines are regulated by the FDA using different methods than those used to regulate prescription medicines, and this difference has important implications for their safety and efficacy in pediatrics. Prescription medicines undergo extensive animal and human testing—actual use studies—prior to entering the commercial marketplace and becoming available for prescribing by physicians. Actual use testing is not required for OTC drug products. Instead, the active ingredients contained in OTC drug products are regulated by drug "monographs." Drug monographs are developed for therapeutic categories of medicines, such as the category of medicines for pain (acetaminophen, ibuprofen).

In 1972, the FDA began one of its most extensive projects, referred to as the OTC Drug Review, by evaluating the safety and efficacy of all active ingredients in these therapeutic categories. This process is ongoing and has not yet been completed. It is estimated that more than 100,000 OTC products are available today, with approximately several hundred different active ingredients contained in these products. Product active ingredients are grouped into more than 80 different therapeutic categories. OTC drug products containing active ingredients determined to be unsafe or ineffective during the Drug Review process have been removed from the marketplace and are no longer available.

How do these regulatory differences between OTC and prescription medicines relate to pediatrics? And what are the implications for giving OTC medicines to your child? For one thing, dose recommendations for children listed on most OTC drug products have been developed by extrapolation of adult doses, which involves reducing doses by percentages based on an adult's weight (for example, 25 percent of an adult drug dose for a child who weighs 25 percent of what an adult weighs). We now know that this method is not accurate and does not reflect the numerous differences between an infant or child's body as compared to an adult's body. This is well illustrated by the use of OTC cough and cold drug products in infants and children (see chapter 1 and below for more about this) and their potential dangers. Thus, although OTC drug products are generally regarded as safe enough to use for self-diagnosis and self-treatment by adults (meaning that a physician's prescription is not needed), their use in the pediatric population may not be as similarly safe and effective.

Appropriate Use and Potential Problems

Over the past five years the instructions for using OTC liquid drug products for children have improved, and consequently these medications are easier to use. In 2011 the FDA published specific guidelines for pharmaceutical manufacturers of OTC liquid drug products. The national trade organization representing OTC drug product manufacturers, the Consumer Healthcare Products Association, released similar recommendations at about the same time. Prior to the publication of these guidelines, an important study was published in the pediatric medical literature in 2010. Researchers in this study evaluated 200 top-selling pediatric liquid OTC drug products and concluded that the vast majority of them contained numerous types of confusing and problematic dosing directions that could easily lead parents to make dosing errors when administering the medications to their children. These potentially problematic dosing directions included, for example, lack of inclusion of a dosing device with the product, inconsistent and confusing dosing directions, and markings on differing parts of the product and packaging, among others.

After release of guidelines by the FDA and industry trade group, another study published by different researchers evaluated pediatric OTC liquid drug products in a similar manner. These researchers concluded that most products had improved and were largely adhering to these guidelines. However, some products were not sufficiently improved, and the potential for parents to easily make mistakes when using them remained. For example, some pediatric OTC liquid drug products may still be using "teaspoonful" or "tablespoonful" as the measurement in dosing directions.

In 2015, the American Academy of Pediatrics and several other major medical organizations recommended that liquid medicines not be dosed with "teaspoonful" or "tablespoonful" measurement directions, and that mL (milliliter) be used instead (see chapter 2 for more information on dosing). Although many OTC liquid drug products are now less likely to be administered incorrectly, the potential remains. As a parent, you should be aware of the possibility of dosing errors with OTC liquid products.

Because OTC medicines can be easily purchased from numerous sources without the benefit of instruction or advice from a physician or pharmacist, the FDA has recently instituted changes to improve product label directions. All OTC drug products are now required to contain standardized "Drug Facts" information (figure 3.1). All OTC drug product labels will provide information in the following categories:

- Active ingredient
- Uses
- Warnings
- Ask a doctor before use if you have . . .
- Ask a doctor or pharmacist before use if you are taking . . .
- When using this product . . .

- Directions
- Other information
- Inactive ingredients

These standardized and simplified label directions should allow parents to use OTC products appropriately while minimizing administration errors.

You will more likely choose and administer safe and effective OTC liquid drug products for your child when you keep the following points in mind:

- Use your child's weight, rather than age, when determining the appropriate dose.
- Use caution when choosing a product with more than one active ingredient. The extra ingredients may not benefit your child, and they may even cause adverse effects.
- Use only the dosing device that comes with the product package. Errors are more likely to occur if you substitute another measuring device.
- Read the label. Be sure to carefully read the Drug Facts to make sure the OTC product is considered safe and effective for your child.
- Be aware that some OTC pediatric drug products should *not* be given to children. Even though their availability may suggest otherwise, some OTC drug products, such as antidiarrheal medications, may not be safe and effective for children.

Treating Common Childhood Illnesses
FEVER

Treating a fever in infants and children is the top reason parents and other caregivers reach for OTC medicines. You likely have given acetaminophen (Tylenol) or ibuprofen (Motrin, Advil) to your child on numerous occasions. Fever is the most common concern when parents call their pediatrician, and it is a major reason why

Drug Facts

Active ingredient (in each tablet)   **Purpose**
Chlorpheniramine maleate 2 mg .... Antihistamine

Uses   temporarily relieves these symptoms due to hay fever or other upper respiratory allergies:
■ sneezing   ■ runny nose   ■ itchy, watery eyes   ■ itchy throat

Warnings

Ask a doctor before use if you have
■ glaucoma   ■ a breathing problem such as emphysema or chronic bronchitis
■ trouble urinating due to an enlarged prostate gland

Ask a doctor or pharmacist before use if you are taking tranquilizers or sedatives

When using this product
■ You may get drowsy   ■ avoid alcoholic drinks
■ alcohol, sedatives, and tranquilizers may increase drowsiness
■ be careful when driving a motor vehicle or operating machinery
■ excitability may occur, especially in children

If pregnant or breast-feeding, ask a health professional before use.
Keep out of reach of children. In case of overdose, get medical help or contact a Poison Control Center right away.

Directions

adults and children 12 years and over	take 2 tablets every 4 to 6 hours; not more than 12 tablets in 24 hours
children 6 years to under 12 years	take 1 tablet every 4 to 6 hours; not more than 6 tablets in 24 hours
children under 6 years	ask a doctor

Other Information   store at 20-25° C (68-77° F)   ■ protect from excessive moisture

Inactive ingredients   D&C yellow no. 10, lactose, magnesium stearate, microcrystalline cellulose, pregelatinized starch

3.1. Example of a "Drug Facts" medicine label. US Department of Health and Human Services, US Food and Drug Administration, fda.gov

infants and children are taken to acute care clinics and hospital emergency departments.

Fortunately, the vast majority of fevers are not dangerous to your child. Many parents harbor "fever phobia," a fear of fever that is often not based in medical reality. The phrase "fever phobia" was coined in 1980 by Dr. Barton Schmitt, the author of a published study that surveyed parents about fever and its effects. Dr. Schmitt found that many parents' concerns and actions about fever did not match medical science. For example, many parents believed that a fever could damage an infant's or child's brain. And some parents would administer acetaminophen or ibuprofen to reduce a fever even when their child appeared comfortable. Several other recently published surveys of parents' thoughts about fever show similar findings: the bottom line is that parents often over-treat their children with regard to fever.

The body temperature many parents consider to be a fever is often not evaluated as a fever by a health care professional. Medically, a normal body temperature is defined as between 97.8°F and 100.3°F, and a fever is defined as a body temperature of 100.4°F (38.0°C) or higher. These published surveys have found that while many parents would consider a specific body temperature to be high for their child, pediatricians would not, and they would not diagnose a fever at that body temperature. An elevated body temperature is not harmful unless a person has very high temperatures, greater than about 106°F, for a prolonged period. This occurs very rarely in children with an infection. Higher body temperatures, temperatures above 105°F to 106°F, can occur with hyperthermia or heat stroke, but these conditions are rare in children.

A fever is not an illness per se but a *symptom* of an illness or medical condition. Pediatricians are most concerned about the *cause* of the fever, and they consider the actual body temperature as less important. Studies and surveys have found that parents are often most focused upon, and concerned with, their child's actual body temperature. From a medical science perspective, fever is an indication that the child's immune system is active and functioning normally to combat the cause of fever, which most commonly results from a viral or bacterial infection. Many published studies of laboratory animals with fever have shown that suppressing a fever increased the likelihood of the animals dying from the infection that was causing the fever. So, a strong argument can be made that fever is a beneficial response to infection.

National guidelines on the treatment of fever have been published by the American Academy of Pediatrics. These guidelines state that the primary goal of treating fever "should be to improve the child's overall comfort rather than focus on the normalization of body temperature." Certainly all parents would like their ill child to be comfortable and feel better, but reducing a child's body temperature to 98.6°F is not necessary to achieve his or her comfort. Acetaminophen and ibuprofen—antipyretic medicines—have benefits, such as improving comfort and allowing your child to return to normal eating, drinking, and sleeping behaviors. Some parents may believe that treating fever and decreasing body temperature reduces the duration and severity of the underlying condition producing the fever. No scientific evidence supports this for the majority of children. A decrease in body temperature can benefit some children with certain specific chronic diseases or severe illnesses by reducing metabolic complications of the illness, but these conditions are uncommon.

When your infant or child develops a fever, you may need to call your pediatrician. When you speak with your pediatrician's office, they likely will want to know your child's temperature and how you measured it. Depending upon your child's age, underlying medical conditions, and other symptoms, the pediatrician may recommend that you bring your child into his or her office or to the hospital emergency department. However, this is often not necessary, and you may be able to treat your child at home, with careful observation for worsening symptoms. Your pediatrician will ask you about your child's activities, behavior, and eating and drinking. Infants and children with a fever often do not eat and drink as much as they normally do, and they can quickly become dehydrated. Young infants, about 6 months of age and younger, should be very carefully observed, as they can become ill more quickly than older infants or children.

A normal dose of acetaminophen or ibuprofen will likely lower your child's body temperature by about 2 or 3°F. So if your child has a fever of 103°F to 104°F, acetaminophen or ibuprofen will decrease the temperature to about 100°F or 101°F, and not 98.6°F. But this temperature reduction will likely allow your child to feel better, which is the goal of treatment. Focus on how your child feels and the activities or other symptoms you discuss with your pediatrician; don't focus on the actual body temperature.

Either acetaminophen (Tylenol) or ibuprofen (Motrin, Advil) can be used to treat your child's fever. They are both effective and safe for infants and children when used appropriately. There are some differences between them, however, that may be important for your child. Your pediatrician will offer guidance. The most important point to understand when using either acetaminophen or ibuprofen is not which product to use. Rather, the key considerations are to give an appropriate dose to your child, not to give this dose too often, and to use your child's comfort and activity, not body temperature, as a guide to help you decide if further doses should be given.

Table 3.1 compares features of acetaminophen and ibuprofen. Note that the dose differs between the two, and that ibuprofen can be given less often since its duration for lowering fever is about two hours longer. Also note that ibuprofen is not recommended for children younger than 6 months, as it has not been well studied and tested in these younger ages. Weight-based doses for acetaminophen and ibuprofen are listed in the table as well. Doses based on your child's weight are most accurate, although dosing by your child's age can be also be used. For example, dosing by age is listed on the bottle and packaging of infants' and children's liquid Tylenol and Motrin products. When you determine a weight-based or age-based dose for your child, always use the dosing device (oral syringe or dosing cup) that comes with the product, and use the closest appropriate volume marking on the device, such as 2.5 mL, 5 mL, 7.5 mL, and so on.

Ibuprofen is more likely to produce adverse effects to an infant or child's kidneys as compared to acetaminophen. This may occur if your child is dehydrated or has other medical conditions that your pediatrician will discuss with you. Several studies have evaluated the potential benefit of treating fever with acetaminophen and ibuprofen combined, or by alternating doses of acetaminophen and ibuprofen. These studies have not demonstrated a clear advantage

Table 3.1 Acetaminophen and ibuprofen for fever

	Acetaminophen*	Ibuprofen
Dose	• 4½–6½ mg per pound, every 4–6 hours when needed • do not give more than 5 times in 24 hours	• 2½–4 mg per pound, every 6–8 hours when needed • do not give more than 4 times in 24 hours
Age	• any age*	• 6 months of age and older
Duration of fever reduction	• 4–6 hours	• 6–8 hours
Dosage forms available for infants and children	• infants' and children's liquid—both contain 160 mg per 5 mL • "junior" chewable tablets—160 mg per tablet	• infants' liquid—50 mg per 1.25 mL • children's liquid—100 mg per 5 mL • "junior" chewable tablets—100 mg per tablet

*Although acetaminophen can be given to young infants, speak with your pediatrician before administering, especially to infants younger than 2 months.

to giving acetaminophen and ibuprofen together or by alternating doses. The guidelines published by the American Academy of Pediatrics discussed above do not recommend alternating or combining doses of acetaminophen and ibuprofen, as it may be confusing or cause more adverse effects than using either acetaminophen or ibuprofen alone.

I tell parents that acetaminophen is a very safe and effective drug to treat fever when it is used appropriately, which means giving correct doses and not giving it too often. However, acetaminophen can be dangerous when an excessive amount is given or when it is given too frequently, which can be toxic to the liver and lead to liver failure, which can be fatal. Many case reports have been published in the literature describing this danger. Risk factors for administering toxic amounts of acetaminophen in these case reports include dosing errors, such as accidentally measuring too much or determining too large of a dose when using liquid acetaminophen products, or giving acetaminophen doses too often. Some of these case reports have described parents accidentally giving their child an adult dosage form of acetaminophen, and consequently an excessive dose. Other scenarios that have occurred involved giving acetaminophen inadvertently from several different OTC medicines, such as giving separate OTC drug products for colds and for fever, all of which contained acetaminophen, without realizing that the overdosing with acetaminophen was occurring.

A stroll down the "cough/cold" and "pain" aisles of your local pharmacy will highlight the vast array of different OTC drug products you can purchase to treat your child's cold or fever. It can be bewildering (and potentially dangerous) deciding which product is best for your child. Most OTC pediatric drug products for cold symptoms that contain several active ingredients will list acetaminophen in yellow highlighted print on the packaging box or bottle if it is one of the active ingredients. If your child has a common cold and a fever, be cautious about giving a multi-ingredient OTC cold product in addition to another OTC product with acetaminophen just for fever.

HOW TO CALCULATE A CORRECT AMOUNT OF FEVER MEDICINE TO GIVE AN INFANT OR CHILD

Here is an example of how to give oral acetaminophen and ibuprofen correctly to an infant with a fever who is uncomfortable.

Example: *Your 10-month-old infant son has a fever of 102.5°F and weighs 22 pounds, or 10 kilograms (kg). You have spoken with your child's pediatrician, and she recommends giving acetaminophen or ibuprofen orally.*

ACETAMINOPHEN (TYLENOL OR GENERIC)

1. How much acetaminophen should I give?

- By weight → 10 to 15 mg per kg or 4.5–6.5 mg per pound = **100–150 mg**
- By age from medication box → "Ask a doctor" → the doctor's office will also tell you to give 100–150 mg.

2. What type of acetaminophen should I use?

Two types of liquid acetaminophen products are available in pharmacies—Infants' and Children's. They both contain liquid acetaminophen in the same strength and concentration, 160 mg per 5 mL. They differ, however, by the dose measuring device that comes with each package. The Infants' product comes with a dosing syringe for measuring smaller volume amounts, and the Children's product comes with a dosage cup for measuring larger volume amounts. The Infants' product is best to use for a 10-month-old infant. The Children's product is best used for children about 2 years of age and older.

3. How should I measure out the amount to give?

Let's use the Infants' acetaminophen product as an example. The next step is to determine how much liquid medicine, or the volume, to measure out. The dosing syringe from the Infants' acetaminophen box has four markings on it: *(continued)*

- **1.25 mL** (equivalent to 40 mg, although it is not stated on the syringe)
- **2.5 mL** (equivalent to 80 mg, although it is not stated on the syringe)
- **3.75 mL** (equivalent to 120 mg, although it is not stated on the syringe)
- **5 mL** (equivalent to 160 mg, although it is not stated on the syringe)

The 3.75 mL marking, or 120 mg, is in the range of 100 to 150 mg calculated for your 10-month-old infant son. Pediatricians' offices refer to dose charts when you call, but you can calculate a dose by yourself. Liquid acetaminophen is 160 mg per 5 mL which equals 32 mg per mL. A dose of 100–150 mg = 3.1–4.7 mL. A dose of 3.75 mL is within this range and easiest and most accurately measured out by the markings on the acetaminophen product syringe. As you can see, determining an accurate dose for your child's weight can be a bit tricky or somewhat difficult. Your pharmacist will be able to help you with these calculations over the phone, if necessary.

4. How often should I give acetaminophen?

Acetaminophen can be given every 4 to 6 hours as needed. Do not give more than 5 doses in a 24-hour period.

5. How do I know if acetaminophen is helping?

Watch your child's comfort level. He should begin feeling better within 30 to 60 minutes of receiving a dose of acetaminophen. Don't focus too much on his temperature, as it may not come down to 98.6°F. If your son's temperature comes down to 99.5°F, and he seems to feel better, then you know that the acetaminophen has helped. Keep in mind that acetaminophen will typically lower a child's temperature by 2° to 3°F, which would be 99.5°F to 100.5°F for your son. Improving your child's comfort, not lowering his temperature to 98.6°F, is the goal of using acetaminophen and treating fever.

IBUPROFEN (MOTRIN, ADVIL, OR A GENERIC BRAND)

1. How much ibuprofen should I give?

- By weight → 5–10 mg per kg, or 2.5–4 mg per pound
  = 50–100 mg
- By age from Infants' ibuprofen medication box:
  - 18–23 pounds → 1.875 mL (3rd line on dropper) or 75 mg
  - 6–11 months → 1.25 mL (2nd line on dropper) or 50 mg
- Notice that different doses are given by age and weight. Both doses are correct, but 75 mg is in the middle of the dose range and is more likely to be effective, as 50 mg is on the low end of the dose range.

2. What type of ibuprofen should I use?

Ibuprofen is available as Infants' and Children's liquid products, as is acetaminophen, but an important difference is ibuprofen Infants' and Children's products differ in concentration, or strength: the Infants' product is *twice as concentrated*—40 mg per mL, as compared to 20 mg per mL for the Children's product. To decrease the amount or volume of liquid medicine to give to your infant, it is best to use the Infants' product.

3. How should I measure out the amount to give?

- **0.625 mL** (equivalent to 25 mg, although it is not stated on the syringe)
- **1.25 mL** (equivalent to 50 mg, although it is not stated on the syringe)
- **1.875 mL** (equivalent to 75 mg, although it is not stated on the syringe)

The third line on the syringe is 75 mg (1.875 mL). This dose is easy to measure and is likely to help your son, as the dose is in the middle of the dose range for your son's weight.

(continued)

4. How often should I give ibuprofen?

Ibuprofen can be given every 6 to 8 hours, but do not give more than 4 doses in a 24-hour period. Notice that ibuprofen lasts 2 to 4 hours longer than acetaminophen, which can be an advantage, especially at night.

5. How do I know if ibuprofen is helping?

Watch your child's comfort level. He should begin feeling better within 30 to 60 minutes of receiving a dose of ibuprofen. Don't focus too much on his temperature, as it may not come down to 98.6°F. If your son's temperature comes down to 99.5°F and he feels better, ibuprofen has helped. Keep in mind that ibuprofen will typically lower a child's temperature by 2° to 3°F, which would be 99.5°F to 100.5°F for your son. Improving your child's comfort, and not lowering his temperature to 98.6°F, is the goal of using ibuprofen and treating fever.

With this example, you may have noticed that it can be easy to make a mistake when trying to determine what dose of acetaminophen or ibuprofen to give your infant or child, what product to use, and how to measure out the correct dose. Don't hesitate to ask your pharmacist or pediatrician for help if you are not sure. Don't guess.

COUGHS AND COLDS

The common cold occurs more frequently in the pediatric population than in the adult population. In fact, infants and children will suffer between six and ten colds each year. With a typical cold producing symptoms of congestion, mild fever, cough, and throat irritation or discomfort for up to ten days, and the possibility of up to ten colds per year, it may seem that your infant or child is nearly continuously ill. When your child has a cold, he or she likely sleeps less, which means that you also sleep less. Parents want their child to feel better, and it becomes tempting to give an OTC drug product to relieve these symptoms. Multi-ingredient OTC cough/cold products contain a variety of active ingredient medicines, most commonly combinations of medicines to treat cough, nasal congestion, antihistamines (supposedly to reduce a runny nose), and perhaps acetaminophen or ibuprofen for fever.

Until about ten years ago, many OTC drug products were available to treat colds in infants and younger children, and these products were advertised and marketed specifically for treating infants and younger children. In 2008, upon recommendations from the FDA and additional voluntary changes from OTC product manufacturers, package labeling and instructions for OTC cough/cold products were changed to read, "Do not use in children under the age of 4 years." Despite their previous availability for these young ages, and their continued availability for children 4 years of age and older, there are no data from clinical studies demonstrating that cough/cold products effectively and safely treat cold symptoms in infants and children. Instead, many published studies and summary reviews of these studies have shown that cough/cold products do not reduce symptoms of the common cold in infants and children, and they can be dangerous to use.

Yet many of these products remain available for purchase. If clinical studies have shown that these products are not effective and safe in children, why do they continue to be available as OTC products? The answer relates to the difference in effectiveness of OTC cough/cold products in children as compared to adults.

The active drug ingredients in OTC cough/cold products have shown some benefit in clinical studies of adults, and due to a lack of similar studies in children, it was assumed over 40 years ago, when OTC drug ingredients began to be formally evaluated, that cough/cold ingredients would have similar benefits in children. Pediatric doses were extrapolated from adult doses based solely on body weight, which is an inaccurate method to determine safe and effective drug doses for infants and children.

Although no data from clinical studies have demonstrated that OTC cough/cold products are effective in infants and children younger than 12 years of age, information has accumulated over the past 40 years showing that these products can be dangerous, and even fatal. From 2004 to 2005 an estimated 1,519 children younger than 2 years of age, as reported by the FDA, were treated in hospital emergency departments for adverse effects, including overdoses, associated with cough and cold drug products. Well over 100 deaths of infants and young children have been described in published reports where OTC cough/cold products were the sole cause or important contributive causes.

Although several doses of pediatric OTC cough/cold products are unlikely to be toxic, these reports have described scenarios where the products were used inappropriately by administration of doses too large, doses given too frequently, doses measured inaccurately (too much liquid), or administration of similar active ingredient medicines given from numerous OTC products resulting in accumulative large doses. These mistakes were easily made by parents, considering the difficulty in accurately measuring out small liquid doses and a desire for the medicines to help (as many people mistakenly believe, when it comes to medicine, that more is better). Thus, the FDA is continuing to review the effectiveness and availability of OTC cough/cold products for children older than 4 years, and new regulations may be issued on their use in the near future. It is best not to give an OTC product marketed for cough and cold symptoms to your child if he or she is younger than 12 years of age.

Your child may also develop a cough from a cold, and this can be troublesome especially at night, reducing sleep. Many OTC drug products are marketed for cough (antitussive), as single-ingredient products or as part of multi-ingredient cough/cold products. The most common antitussive ingredient in OTC products is dextromethorphan, found in products such as Robitussin DM. In 1997 the Committee on Drugs of the American Academy of Pediatrics published recommendations on the treatment of cough and stated that there are no data from clinical studies demonstrating that dextromethorphan effectively and safely reduces cough in children. Similar to other OTC cough/cold drug products, dextromethorphan has remained available in OTC products likely because it can be effective in adults, and this efficacy had been assumed years ago to be similar in children. However, children are not small adults, and this assumption is not accurate.

Two well-done studies have recently been published describing the beneficial effects of honey in treating children's coughs. These studies evaluated various types of honey (such as buckwheat honey) given at bedtime, and demonstrated that cough was reduced. It is not known if other types of honey, such as clover honey (amber in color, and widely available in grocery stores), are as effective. Doses of honey given in these studies were ½ to 1 teaspoonful (2.5 to 5 mL) for children 1 to 5 years of age, 1 teaspoonful (5 mL) for ages 6 to 11 years, and 2 teaspoonsful (10 mL) for older children. Other than a single bedtime dose, how often these doses can be repeated was not studied, although every 3 to 4 hours as needed seems reasonable. Note that "teaspoonful" is described here, although I discussed in chapter 2 that current recommendations state not to use teaspoons or tablespoons as liquid medication measuring devices. This is still true. The accuracy of dosing honey, a food item, for cough is not nearly as important as it is for liquid medicines. Because honey may contain bacterial spores that can be dangerous to infants younger than 1 year, *honey should not be given to any infant younger than 12 months of age.*

Codeine is another drug that has been used to treat cough for many years; it continues to be available in some states without a prescription. Although codeine remains available in some OTC cough products, and is also included in several prescription liquid cough medicines, it should not be used as a cough suppressant in children. Evidence has accumulated over the past ten years demonstrating that codeine can produce a significant decrease in breathing in some infants and children. More than 20 cases of fatal respiratory depression have been documented in infants and children.

Codeine does not have any pharmacologic effect in the body and it is chemically altered (metabolized) by the liver to form morphine and another active metabolite. We have learned that the amount of morphine produced from codeine liver metabolism can vary widely from person to person. Some individuals may convert codeine to a lot of morphine, while others may convert codeine to much less morphine. Morphine is a potent inhibitor of respiration, or breathing. This concept that inherited genetic differences may affect how an individual responds to a drug is termed *pharmacogenetics*, and is an active area of drug research. For many years we have known that no studies exist to support the use of codeine as an effective cough suppressant in children, and in 1997 the American Academy of Pediatrics recommended *not* to use codeine for this purpose. In 2015 the FDA similarly recommended that codeine not be used to treat cough in children. In 2016, the American Academy of Pediatrics published additional warnings on the dangers of administering codeine to infants and children, recommending that its use for all purposes in children, including cough and pain, be limited or stopped.

So what can you do to help your infant or child with a cough or cold feel better? As with all of the illnesses discussed in this book, an important first step when treating your child is to speak with your pediatrician. Some severe infections may initially appear to be a cold or fever in your child, but can quickly progress to a more serious illness. Your pediatrician will talk with you and monitor your child for changes. If your child has a common cold, consider using some of the treatments described below. They are likely to be beneficial and much safer than OTC multi-ingredient cough/cold drug products.

The common cold can produce many annoying and troubling symptoms in infants and children. A stuffy or runny nose can be especially troublesome to infants younger than 6 months of age because they have difficulty breathing through their mouths like older children can. Not being able to breathe while feeding can be especially distressing for a young infant. Several simple remedies are likely to help. Bulb suctioning devices for removing nasal mucus from infants and young children can clear nasal passages. A similar device is a nasal aspirator that allows you, through attached but separate tubing, to use your inspiratory breathing force to suck out congestion from your infant's nose. Your infant's nasal contents do not come into contact with your lips or mouth, but are collected into a separate chamber. An example is BabyComfyNose nasal aspirator (available online for about $15).

Other products that relieve symptoms and are likely to be safer than OTC cough and cold products include the following:

- Saline solution drops or sprays for nasal stuffiness help to loosen dried and plugged nasal mucus and to decrease nasal congestion and improve breathing.
- Cold water humidifiers (vaporizers) humidify the air in your child's room, which will decrease nasal congestion.
- Honey for cough, for ages 12 months and older.

DIARRHEA

Diarrhea, called acute gastroenteritis, is another common reason that parents call their pediatrician or bring their child into a pediatrician's office. The majority of diarrheal episodes in infants and children are due to viral causes, often referred to as "stomach viruses" or "stomach bugs," and they usually self-resolve with time. Parents often focus on trying to stop their child's diarrhea, but a more appropriate focus is to prevent the dehydration that often results from excessive loss of fluid.

Although several OTC products are marketed to treat children with diarrhea, *they should not be used in children*. These products include Imodium AD, Kaopectate, and Pepto-Bismol. Imodium AD contains loperamide, which is an antimotility drug. It slows down the movement of fecal material through the intestinal tract. While this may seem to be beneficial for stopping diarrhea, loperamide has been known to cause severe slowing of intestinal movement and intestinal blockage in some children, resulting in death. Kaopectate and Pepto-Bismol both contain the drug bismuth subsalicylate, which is chemically similar to aspirin and may result in dangerous adverse effects when given to children. These medicines may be helpful when taken by adults with diarrhea, but as I have stated often throughout this book, children are not small adults.

If your pediatrician assesses that your child is dehydrated, you will likely be told to give some type of oral rehydration solution (ORS). Common brands of ORS widely available in pharmacies and grocery stores are Pedialyte and Enfalyte. Pedialyte and other ORS products contain a specifically balanced mixture of glucose, sodium, potassium, and additional electrolytes. These body chemicals are lost in diarrheal fluid and need to be replaced to rehydrate your child and prevent further dehydration. Infants and young children can quickly become dehydrated from diarrhea and may need to be hospitalized if dehydration is severe.

It may be tempting to give your child water, juice, or other liquids. These should not be used, however, as they do not contain the balanced mixture of glucose and electrolytes that your child needs. Juices can increase diarrhea and fluid loss because they contain a lot of sugar and can produce additional fluid loss from the intestines. Unfortunately, many children dislike the taste of the commonly available ORS products. Pedialyte and other oral rehydration solutions are available in flavors (grape, bubblegum, mixed fruit, and others) and these probably have a better taste than the unflavored Pedialyte. Chilling Pedialyte in the refrigerator will also improve the taste. For older children, ORS products are available as freezer pops. It is best to give only small amounts (about 1 ounce) of ORS, but give it frequently, about every 10 to 15 minutes. If you allow your child to drink as much as he or she wants, the fluids will likely be vomited back up. This happened to me when my son was about 4 years old and suffering from diarrhea. I gave him too much fruit Pedialyte, a bright red liquid, and he vomited it up after a few minutes all over the white t-shirt I was wearing!

Complementary and Alternative Medicines

The term complementary and alternative medicine (CAM) is used to describe a group of diverse medical and health care therapies and practices that are not considered to be part of conventional, or western, medicine. CAM is also referred to as holistic or integrative medicine. There are many forms of CAM, including herbal medicines, probiotics, homeopathy, acupuncture, hypnosis, meditation, and yoga, among many others. Some of these therapies, such as herbals and probiotics, are taken orally as capsules, tablets, or as powder formulations. Herbal medicines (such as echinacea), probiotics, and melatonin are products commonly available in many pharmacies and can be purchased without a prescription. The term "supplements" is also used to describe these alternative orally administered products. The FDA defines dietary supplements as herbal products, vitamins, minerals, and other dietary substances.

CAM therapies are commonly used in the pediatric population. The National Health Interview Survey, a large survey of representative US households conducted in 2012 (17,321 interviews) by the Centers for Disease Control and Prevention (CDC), evaluated CAM use in children 4 to 17 years of age. This survey revealed that CAM therapies were used by 11.6 percent of children. CAM therapies are used to treat anxiety, musculoskeletal conditions, recurrent headaches, and colds in both children and adults. Parents who use CAM therapies themselves are most likely to use them with their children. The supplements most commonly used in 2012 by children 4 to 17 years of age were fish oil, melatonin, probiotics, and echinacea. Some parents give fish oil to their children with attention deficit–hyperactivity disorder (ADHD) (see chapter 4 for more on this topic). Melatonin, probiotics, and echinacea are discussed below.

Regulation and Manufacture

It is important to have an appreciation for the significant differences between CAM supplements and traditional prescription and OTC medicines. Laws regulating the manufacture and evaluation of product safety and efficacy of traditional medicines and CAM therapies are notably different. These laws are significantly less stringent for CAM therapies. As discussed in chapter 1, prescription medicines must be demonstrated to be safe and effective in animal and human clinical studies before they are approved by the FDA and made available to the public. For a typical prescription drug, documentation of product safety and efficacy entails thousands of pages of data and information that are submitted to FDA officials for careful review. Although the regulations and processes for labeling of OTC drug product ingredients are not as in-depth as those for prescription medicines, the FDA has been extensively reviewing all categories of OTC drug product ingredients for safety and efficacy for over 40 years, and this process is continuing.

In 1994, Congress approved the Dietary Supplement Health and Education Act (DSHEA), which regulates the manufacture and availability of CAM supplements. This law strives to reach a balance between consumer access to CAM products and the ability of the FDA to remove dangerous products from public availability when necessary. However, it is not nearly as powerful or stringent as the laws regulating the safety and efficacy of prescription and OTC medicines, a point that is important to appreciate and keep firmly in mind.

Under DSHEA, supplement manufacturers do not have to demonstrate stringent purity and potency standards as do pharmaceutical manufacturers of prescription and OTC medicines, nor do they have to prove safety and efficacy from human clinical studies prior to marketing and public availability. There are thousands of supplement manufacturers, and it becomes very difficult for the FDA to carefully inspect supplement manufacturing facilities to ensure that appropriate procedures are used to safely produce supplement products. The FDA has reported that supplement products are sometimes being manufactured in residential basements or laboratories the size of a bathroom.

The manufacturers of supplements evaluate the product safety, purity, and potency by the honor system. They do not conduct stringent human testing as is done with prescription and OTC medicines. As you may imagine, this invites problems. Consumers assume that supplements are safe and contain the ingredients listed on the product label, but there is no guarantee.

And what about efficacy? Although supplements are not rigorously tested for effectiveness, manufacturers cannot claim false statements of efficacy either. A common statement found on supplement product labels regarding potential benefits of the product is, "This statement has not been evaluated by the Food and Drug Administration. This product is not intended to diagnose, treat, cure, or prevent disease." Thus, when you buy a supplement product, there is often no proof that the product will effectively do what the packaging label or its advertising claims, or that the product actually contains the amount of active ingredient stated on the label.

Some conventional medicines, such as digoxin and aspirin, were originally discovered and synthesized from natural plant sources. Digoxin, derived from the foxglove plant, is a drug used for some heart problems. Aspirin (acetylsalicylic acid) is made from willow tree leaves. Clearly some plants have natural medicinal properties. However, there is a significant difference between the theoretical and potential medical value of a plant and the real, proven therapeutic benefits of its chemical components, and in what parts of the plant the medicinal chemicals are found.

The bottles and packaging of supplement products on display at the local pharmacy have a professional appearance, similar to OTC products. It is easy for a consumer to be lulled into thinking that herbal and supplement products are as safe and effective as OTC medicines, such as acetaminophen or ibuprofen. However, this may be a false assumption. The specific plant components that are safe and effective to use by humans, including the exact amount, is best determined through rigorous testing by the standards and procedures used for studying conventional medicines. This testing often is not done with herbal products, and it is not currently required by law.

Some supplement products include wording like "all natural" or "natural" on the product bottle and packaging. It is easy to understand why someone might assume that because an herbal or other supplement product is "natural," it must therefore be safe, perhaps even safer than prescription medicines. However, this assumption may not be accurate. There are recent reports providing evidence that supplements can be dangerous. The FDA has received over 6,000 reports of adverse effects, including more than 1,000 considered to be serious, and 92 deaths from supplements in recent years. Most recently, the FDA issued a "warning" about homeopathic teething tablets and gels available in at least one major national pharmacy chain after seizures and breathing difficulties occurred with their use.

Because supplement products are not rigorously evaluated for purity and potency, they may not always contain what is stated on the package label, and incidents of these inaccurate labels have recently been reported. In 2015 the New York Attorney General's office evaluated several popular herbal products for their content and found that the majority did not contain the active ingredients listed on the product's label. These products were sold at major national retailers, such as Target, Walgreens, Walmart, and GNC. Instead of the stated active ingredients, many of the products tested contained rice, houseplants, carrots, asparagus, beans, or peas. Some even contained peanuts, a potent allergen for some children. Although these products have since been removed from store shelves or reformulated to more accurately contain labeled ingredients, it is likely, since supplement manufacturing is not strongly regulated, that other products similarly do not contain what their labels list. Other published studies have included case reports of various herbal products contaminated with lead or potent prescription medicines, with high potential for toxicity when given to children.

Probiotics

Recent studies supported by the federal government's National Institutes of Health have demonstrated that the human body contains up to ten times the number of bacteria, termed the human microbiome, as human cells. We are accustomed to associating bacteria with infection or disease, but many of the ones found in our bodies are termed "good" bacteria, since they aid in essential processes like digestion and maintenance of a healthy immune system. Most of these good bacteria are found in our gastrointestinal tract (where you might find about 500 different species of bacteria). What do these bacteria do for us? Recent studies suggest that they contribute to food digestion, help our immune systems defend against other dangerous types of bacteria, and assist with synthesizing vitamins, among other benefits. When an infant is born, his or her gastrointestinal system contains no bacteria, but immediately after birth it begins to become populated with good bacteria from the mother and the infant's environment. We are beginning to learn and investigate the relationship between alterations in the human microbiome and human diseases.

Probiotics are "live microorganisms that, when administered in adequate amounts, confer a health benefit on the host" (International Scientific Association for Probiotics and Prebiotics, 2014). A prebiotic is "a non-digestible food ingredient that benefits the host by selectively stimulating the favorable growth and/or activity of 1 or more indigenous probiotic bacteria" (American Academy of Pediatrics, 2010). The idea of giving "good" bacteria to humans is not new; it was first suggested over a hundred years ago. Each year medical journals publish hundreds of studies evaluating the benefits of probiotics. Their use in children has increased many fold in recent years. Your local health food store, and pharmacy, likely contains many different probiotic products on their shelves, as capsules, tablets, powder, and liquids. Some infant nutritional formulas also contain probiotics.

Probiotics have been studied for many uses in infants and children, and recent summary reviews and guidelines describing these studies have been published. Not all of these potential uses, however, have been shown by clinical studies to be effective. Benefits demonstrated by clinical studies and accepted by pediatricians include:

- decreasing the amount and frequency of viral diarrhea in otherwise healthy children—probiotics can decrease the amount and frequency of diarrhea by about 1 day, if given early, within 48 hours of the onset of diarrhea; and
- preventing diarrhea associated with using antibiotics— antibiotics can destroy normal good bacteria in the intestines, causing diarrhea.

Other studies have suggested additional benefits of probiotics, although the evidence is not as convincing as it is for the uses above. Studies are continuing, and we may have additional evidence of more probiotic benefits in the near future. Probiotics are considered supplements and some probiotic products may make claims on the package labeling that infer greater benefits than clinical studies have demonstrated. Before giving your child a probiotic product, talk with your pediatrician.

If you and your pediatrician decide that a probiotic will benefit your child, it is important to consider the type of bacteria contained in the product, and the amount, or dose, of the bacteria. Many probiotic products are available, and they differ widely by the specific bacteria and the amount of bacteria contained in them. Clinical studies documenting the benefit of a specific bacterial species of probiotic may not confirm that the same benefits apply to a different bacterial species. Also important is the dose, or the number of bacterial organisms contained in the product. Bacterial species demonstrated to be effective in the studies of viral diarrhea treatment and prevention of antibiotic-associated diarrhea are *Lactobacillus rhamnosus* GG (LGG) and the yeast *Saccharomyces boulardii*. Listed below are specific probiotic products containing an appropriate number of these bacterial and yeast species and likely to be effective:

- Culturelle Kids
- Florastor Kids
- Florajen4Kids

Melatonin

Melatonin is a natural hormone produced in the brain and it functions to help regulate circadian rhythms (distinguishing day and night) and sleep. Melatonin is sold as a supplement to help people sleep and is available in different strengths and dosage forms. As reported in the 2012 National Health Interview Survey of children 4 to 17 years of age, melatonin is among the most commonly used supplements.

Before considering giving melatonin or an OTC drug to help your child sleep, speak with your pediatrician about using good sleep hygiene practices to help your child sleep better. When these steps are implemented, children often do not need a supplement or OTC drug. Good sleep hygiene includes having regular bedtime and wake-up times, avoiding screen time (television, computer use) just before bedtime, and other practical steps.

Studies have shown melatonin to be beneficial to children with attention deficit–hyperactivity disorder (ADHD) and other neurodevelopmental disorders. However, in otherwise healthy children, there are few data from clinical studies to support the use of melatonin to improve sleep. The most appropriate dose and the long-term adverse effects of melatonin use in otherwise healthy children are also not known. Some pediatric references maintain that it is reasonable to try melatonin for a short time if additional help is still needed after implementing good sleep hygiene practices.

A dose of 2 to 3 mg may be tried. Some pediatric experts have expressed concerns about giving a medicine, and a hormone (melatonin is a hormone), to help otherwise healthy children sleep. If you try melatonin, keep your pediatrician informed, and it's best to use it short-term only, no longer than one or two weeks.

Echinacea

Echinacea is a natural herb obtained from parts of the echinacea plant, including the leaves and roots. Because supplements are loosely regulated, herbal products advertised as containing a specific plant, such as echinacea, may contain widely varying amounts of different species of the plant and various parts of the plant. The effectiveness of the supplement depends on these fine points, which can make it quite confusing when trying to choose a specific product from the store shelf.

Echinacea is marketed for the treatment and prevention of the common cold and other upper respiratory tract infections. A relatively large number of studies have been published on echinacea, mostly in adults. Reviews of this information demonstrate that some studies have shown a mild benefit, while other studies have not demonstrated any benefit. The National Center for Complementary and Alternative Medicine, part of the federal government's National Institutes of Health, describes the overall treatment effects of echinacea as "weak." One published study found that echinacea caused an increased risk of rash in children.

I don't recommend that you give your child echinacea until additional studies demonstrating its benefit to children are completed and published. There are several safe treatments you can use to help your child feel better from a cold (see the section on common colds, above), and they are likely safer and more effective than echinacea.

Vitamins

Vitamin products are a big business, as a visit to your pharmacy will demonstrate. It is likely that one entire aisle is dedicated to carrying various types of vitamin products, including multivitamins, separate vitamin products for vitamins B, C, D, and E, and various combinations of these vitamins. Children are the intended market for chewables, gummy vitamins, Flintstones vitamins, and more. Does your child need a vitamin supplement if he or she is a good eater? Would your child benefit from a vitamin supplement if he or she is a picky eater? Do vitamins have adverse effects if too much is given? These are good questions to ask your pediatrician, and I address them below.

The American Academy of Pediatrics states that healthy children who have a well-balanced diet do not need vitamin supplements. Children who do not eat well, are very picky eaters, or have specific diets, such as vegetarian with few dairy products, may benefit from a vitamin supplement. If you have such a child, it is best to speak with your pediatrician before purchasing a vitamin supplement. Some diseases and medicines may increase the need for specific vitamins. If your child requires additional vitamins because of a medical condition, your pediatrician will discuss this with you.

It is easy to think of vitamins as natural and safe, but it is possible to have too much of a good thing, with adverse effects. Some vitamins, namely fat-soluble vitamins (A, D, E, and K) remain in parts of the body that have higher concentrations of fat for a significantly longer time than other vitamins, such as water-soluble vitamins (B and C).

Vitamin D has received specific attention recently by the American Academy of Pediatrics. In 2011, the recommended daily allowance (RDA) of vitamin D in pediatrics was raised. A major function of vitamin D is to increase the absorption of calcium and phosphorus from foods, and to increase and support bone function and strength. About one-half of an adult's bone mass is stockpiled during adolescence, and by 18 years of age, we have about nine-tenths of our peak bone mass. Thus, obtaining sufficient quantities of calcium and vitamin D from a good diet are important throughout childhood.

Recent studies have shown that the majority of adolescents do not receive enough calcium through their diet. High amounts of vitamin D are found in many food sources, mostly dairy products, but also in shitake mushrooms and other vegetables (spinach, collards, and broccoli, for example), fatty fish (salmon, tuna, and other fishes), and some supplemented foods, including orange juice and various cereals. Milk is an excellent source of vitamin D. Dairy products, including yogurt, are also great sources of calcium.

Young infants sometimes require a vitamin D supplement. Since human breast milk does not contain an adequate amount of vitamin D, an infant who is sustained entirely on breast milk will need a supplement. If your newborn infant is entirely breastfed or even partially breastfed and partially formula-fed, your pediatrician will likely recommend a vitamin D supplement. All commercial infant formulas contain vitamin D, but an adequate amount of formula has to be consumed to meet daily vitamin D requirements (about 32 ounces of formula a day). Most newborn and young infants consuming formula will still require a daily vitamin D supplement. The current recommended dose of vitamin D is 400 international units (IU) daily for infants until the age of 12 months.

Milk is an excellent source of vitamin D and calcium. However, because the protein in cow's milk is more difficult for infants to digest, and cow's milk does not contain enough iron and other nutrients that young infants need, milk should not be given to infants younger than 12 months of age. However, starting at 12 months, children benefit from drinking milk.

Infants 1 year of age and children up to the age of 18 years require 600 IU of vitamin D daily. If your infant or child is healthy and has a good diet, including food sources high in vitamin D and calcium, especially dairy products, supplemental vitamin or calcium is likely not necessary. Children with certain medical conditions (such as cystic fibrosis) or those who use particular prescription medications may require supplemental vitamin D and calcium. Your pediatrician will discuss this further with you.

How to Choose a Supplement Product

If you and your pediatrician decide that your child may benefit from a probiotic, vitamin, or other supplement, you will need to learn to select carefully. Because supplements are not as stringently regulated for purity, efficacy, and safety as prescription and OTC drug products, you should be aware of several characteristics that indicate if the product is likely to contain what its package label states.

When deciding on a specific product to purchase, be skeptical of words like "natural," "all natural," "certified," or "approved" on the bottle or packaging. These words are meaningless and have no scientific or clinical benefit. There are seals from independent testing organizations that you can look for, however, and these do have some practical meaning and benefit.

- US Pharmacopeia (USP)
- Consumerlab.com
- NSF International

Supplement companies must pay a fee to the testing laboratories to evaluate their products. This testing is typically done one or several times per year. Look for the seal and name of these testing organizations on the product bottle.

One or more of these seals on a supplement product indicates that the product is more likely to contain what is stated on the product label and package, that it was produced using good manufacturing procedures, and that it does not contain other substances that can be dangerous to infants and children (as noted, some supplements recently tested have been found to contain lead, or even prescription medicines, so we know that some products are poorly manufactured).

Although the presence of the seals from the testing organizations indicates that the product is more likely to contain only what is on the product label, it does not imply that the product is therapeutically effective for a specific illness or medical condition, nor that the active ingredients have been proven safe by clinical studies. If your child is receiving any supplement product, be sure to inform your pediatrician and other health care providers. Parents often do not consider a supplement, such as vitamin, herbal product, or probiotic, a "medicine," and they neglect to include it in a list of medications the child is receiving. However, it is important for health care providers to know what your child is receiving, including supplements, because some supplements may interact negatively with prescription or OTC medicines, and their use may affect additional treatment decisions and therapies that your health care provider may consider for your child.

Several reliable and informative Internet sites can help you evaluate specific supplement products to help you decide if your child will benefit from a supplement. These websites are:

- www.usp.org/USPVerified/dietarySupplements
  - website for the U.S. Pharmacopiea
  - lists many products that have been tested
- www.nsf.org
  - website for NSF International, a public health and safety organization

Summary Points for Parents

- The cause of your child's fever is more important than your child's actual body temperature, as fever is not inherently dangerous.

- The goal of treating your child's fever should be to increase comfort and improve eating and drinking, not to lower body temperature to normal.

- Either acetaminophen or ibuprofen can be used to treat your child's fever, with some differences between them.

- When using acetaminophen or ibuprofen, it is important to systematically determine an appropriate dose and measure liquid doses carefully.

- Many OTC drug products for colds contain additional acetaminophen—be careful not to give your child more than one product containing acetaminophen.

- Acetaminophen can be toxic if too much is given.

- OTC drugs for cough and cold are not effective in young children and can be dangerous to use.

- Some remedies, such as saline nasal sprays and honey, can be effectively and safely used to treat your child's cold symptoms.

- When your child has diarrhea, give oral rehydration solutions and not antidiarrheal OTC drug products.

- Complementary and alternative medicine products are not stringently regulated for potency, efficacy, and safety.

- Very little scientific information supports a benefit for use of echinacea or melatonin in children.

- Probiotics may help some children with diarrhea.

- Most children with a good diet do not require supplemental vitamins.

- Infants and some children will benefit from supplemental vitamin D.

- Be careful when choosing a supplement product, and look for products that have been evaluated by testing laboratories.

4

Medicines Used to Treat Depression and Attention Deficit–Hyperactivity Disorder

Depression and attention deficit–hyperactivity disorder (ADHD) are common diagnoses in children and adolescents, and medications are often used to treat these disorders. Within the medical community of physicians and other health care professionals, some controversy surrounds the use of the different antidepressant and stimulant medicines that may be prescribed as part of a treatment plan. These controversies often extend to concerns parents and adolescent patients have, raising questions like these:

- Do antidepressants increase a risk of suicide?
- Are stimulant medicines used to treat ADHD addicting?
- Will stimulant medicines increase the likelihood of a teenager using street drugs or other drugs?

It is not uncommon for parents and adolescents to harbor certain stereotypes or beliefs about antidepressants and stimulants that are not totally medically accurate, and the stigmas attached to these medications can affect your, and your child's or teenager's, desire to use the medicines that are prescribed. In this chapter I discuss how these medicines can be effectively used to treat depression and

ADHD, and I address the issues surrounding these controversies and stigmas in the hope of helping you become more informed about these medicines.

Depression

When you ask someone to picture a person with depression, what probably comes to mind first is an adult, not a child or adolescent. Yet depression commonly occurs in the pediatric population, with up to 9 percent of teenagers fulfilling the criteria to be medically diagnosed with depression at any given time, and up to 25 percent of teens having a history of depression at some time during their adolescence.

Depression in adolescents can appear in numerous ways and can have a significant debilitating effect on the adolescent's life and his or her family's life as well. Symptoms seen in depressed adolescents include:

- depressed mood; irritability and crankiness
- decreased interest in or enjoyment of favored activities, such as sports, video games, or socializing with friends
- insomnia or sleeping more than normal, such as refusing to get out of bed in the morning
- reduced physical activity and movement
- increase in not getting along well with family or friends
- noticeable weight gain or loss
- fatigue and loss of energy
- low self-esteem
- feelings of guilt
- decreased ability to concentrate or make decisions
- worsening academic performance, including an increase in school absence
- recurrent suicidal ideation or behavior

Some of these behaviors may seem to be "normal" for teenagers, and they can be typical, to some extent. However, when a child or adolescent displays many of them, and when they significantly affect the child's or adolescent's life, a medical diagnosis of depression is more likely. If these behaviors occur, they are best evaluated by a physician who can determine if the child or adolescent does indeed have depression. If your teenager is diagnosed with depression, the "good" news is that it likely can be successfully treated with a combination of different approaches, including psychotherapy (counseling) and medicine therapy.

Psychotherapy

If your child or teenager is diagnosed with mild depression, active support by your pediatrician and close monitoring may be tried initially, as many studies have demonstrated that this approach can be effective. If active support and close monitoring by your pediatrician are not helpful, or if moderate or severe depression is diagnosed, psychotherapy, or counseling, will be recommended. Psychotherapy alone can effectively treat moderately severe depression. If additional treatment is needed, antidepressant medicines are given.

Psychotherapy for depression generally entails cognitive behavioral therapy (CBT) or interpersonal therapy (IPT). These therapies are given by trained mental health professionals, such as psychologists, therapists, or counselors. CBT relates to how the child's or teenager's thoughts influence behaviors and feelings, and it targets thoughts and behaviors to improve mood. IPT relates to how interpersonal relationships or problems can affect mood and depression, and how depression can adversely affect interpersonal relationships and problems. Both of these therapies can be effective, and they typically require at least 8 to 12 weeks of treatment for benefits to be noticed.

Antidepressant Medicines

Antidepressant medicines play an important role in the treatment of depression. Guidelines on the treatment of depression have been published by such professional medical organizations as the American Academy of Child and Adolescent Psychiatry and the American Academy of Pediatrics. These guidelines state that antidepressants are best used for moderate or severe depression, and in combination with psychotherapy. Several large, well-done clinical studies have demonstrated that psychotherapy plus antidepressants is more effective than either psychotherapy or antidepressants used alone.

Unfortunately, from the patient's point of view, psychotherapy is often a more difficult treatment to pursue since it requires at least 8 to 12 visits with a counselor or psychologist and may not be fully covered by medical insurance. Antidepressant medicines are easier to use, swallowing just one or more tablets daily, and because most are available generically, they are relatively inexpensive. One of the largest studies of adolescent depression treatment, including more than 400 adolescents ages 12 to 17 years who had moderate or severe depression, compared CBT alone to a combination of CBT and an antidepressant, and to placebo (no active treatment). Of the adolescents receiving combination therapy, 71 percent improved, while 43 percent of those receiving CBT alone improved, 61 percent of those receiving an antidepressant medicine alone improved, and 35 percent of those receiving placebo (no active treatment) improved. This study demonstrates that a combination of psychotherapy and antidepressant medicine is most likely to help an adolescent with depression.

If an antidepressant medicine is recommended for your child or adolescent, your pediatrician or psychiatrist can choose from several different classes of medicines. One class in particular, selective serotonin reuptake inhibitors (SSRIs), is recommended and most commonly used. Serotonin is a neurotransmitter, a chemical that relays messages between nerve cells, and is located throughout our bodies, in blood, the gastrointestinal tract, and in our brain. In the brain, serotonin helps to regulate and control our mood, sleep, and to some extent, our appetite. SSRI medicines increase the amount of serotonin that remains active in our brains, and it is likely by this action that SSRIs help to decrease depression. "Likely" is used here, as researchers and health care professionals are not fully confident that this is how the SSRIs function to treat depression. The chemistry of the brain is complex, and the action of SSRIs in the brain may not be as simple as this.

Other types of antidepressants include tricyclic antidepressants and several other categories of medicines. The tricyclic antidepressants, such as amitriptyline, are much older medicines. These medicines have many more adverse effects than the SSRIs and they can be dangerous if too much is taken. An overdose of these medicines can be used in attempting suicide, so they are often avoided in treating a severely depressed person. The SSRIs are a much safer class of medicines in this respect.

The SSRI class of antidepressant medicines is preferentially recommended by the professional medical organizations discussed above and include the following (generic name followed by trade name):

- fluoxetine (Prozac); ages 8 and older
- escitalopram (Lexapro); ages 12 and older
- citalopram (Celexa)
- paroxetine (Paxil)
- sertraline (Zoloft)
- fluvoxamine (Luvox)
- vilazodone (Viibryd)

As indicated, among the SSRI antidepressants, only fluoxetine and escitalopram are labeled for use by the FDA to treat depression in children and adolescents. (Pediatric use labeling means that these specific antidepressants have been formally studied by a pharmaceutical manufacturer and the FDA has approved their safe and effective use.) Any of the antidepressants listed above can be prescribed by a physician, although the antidepressants with more pediatric use experience are the safer choice.

Fluoxetine (Prozac) has the most evidence for the beneficial treatment of depression in children and adolescents as compared to the other SSRIs, and for this reason it is often described as the first medicine of choice when treating depression in children and adolescents. If fluoxetine (Prozac) or escitalopram (Lexapro) are tried and are not as effective as desired in a child or adolescent, a pediatrician can reasonably prescribe one of the other SSRIs listed above, even though they are not labeled by the FDA for this use. Some pediatric studies have been conducted with these other antidepressants, just not as many as with fluoxetine (Prozac) or escitalopram (Lexapro). Other classes of antidepressants are available and are commonly used to treat depression in adults, including a similar class of medicines, referred to as SNRIs (serotonin–norepinephrine reuptake inhibitors). Commonly used SNRIs include venlafaxine (Effexor) and duloxetine (Cymbalta). We do not have as much experience with clinical studies of these antidepressants in children and adolescents, and thus they are not recommended initially.

As with any medicine, fluoxetine (Prozac) and escitalopram (Lexapro) have adverse effects, although these adverse effects do not prevent most children or adolescents from continuing to take the medicine. Occasionally, however, one or more adverse effects can be a problem and will make it necessary to stop the antidepressant. Common adverse effects from SSRI antidepressants, and what you can do to prevent them from occurring, or lessening their impact, include:

- nausea or upset stomach
  - take with a snack or meal
- headache
  - use acetaminophen (Tylenol) or ibuprofen (Motrin, Advil) as needed; if headaches do occur, they should slowly resolve over 1 to 3 weeks
- feelings of sedation or tiredness
  - take at bedtime

- trouble sleeping
  - take in the morning
- increased sweating
  - use an antiperspirant, or talk with your doctor if troubling
- sexual side effects (decreased libido or impotence)
  - talk with your doctor about trying a different antidepressant
- behavioral activation, including agitation, restlessness, irritability, acting silly, or impulsivity
  - talk with your doctor about trying a different antidepressant

Some of these adverse effects, such as nausea or sedation, may slowly resolve over the first 1 to 3 weeks of treatment. If the adverse effect is too troubling, speak with your pediatrician. Pediatricians or psychiatrists will often start an antidepressant with a low dose for 1 or 2 weeks, and if no or few adverse effects occur, then increase the dose after those first weeks.

As stated throughout this book, every medicine has a potential to cause unwanted adverse effects. It is always important to consider the medicine's benefit-to-risk effects—that is, if the medicine is providing a noticeable benefit in treating the disorder, and the adverse effects are mild and manageable, it seems reasonable to continue the medicine. If the adverse effects are troubling, then the risk of taking the medicine can outweigh the benefit, and it then seems reasonable to try a different medicine.

Common problems that adolescents face when taking antidepressant medicines are listed below, with suggestions for prevention or improvement:

- stopping the antidepressant too soon
  - the SSRI antidepressants require at least 2 to 3 weeks, and often 4 to 6 weeks, to have a noticeable benefit
  - give the antidepressant 4 to 6 weeks before deciding it is not helping
  - positive changes in mood are often not noticeable for 3 to 4 weeks after starting an antidepressant

- missing doses
  - doses of the SSRI antidepressants are normally given once a day; it usually is not important what time of day the antidepressant is taken
  - if the antidepressant causes tiredness, then give it at bedtime, and if it causes your child to feel more awake or active, give it in the morning
  - whatever time of day that suits you and your child is a good time to take the antidepressant, and it is best to take it at about the same time each day
  - if your child misses one dose, the missed dose can be taken up to 12 hours later; for example, if a normal bedtime dose is missed, it can safely be given the next morning, and that same day's bedtime dose can still be given
  - do not take 2 or more doses at the same time
- stopping the antidepressant because your child doesn't believe it is helping, or your child believes it is no longer needed
  - as discussed above, as many as 4 to 6 weeks are often needed for an antidepressant medicine to help
  - family and friends may notice more than your child does that the antidepressant is helping, perhaps in subtle ways
  - it is possible that the antidepressant is not helping, but discuss this with your pediatrician before stopping the medicine; it is important to visit with your pediatrician for follow-up appointments so these concerns and questions can be discussed
- stopping the antidepressant because your child doesn't like taking a medicine to feel "normal"
  - some people do not like to take medicines, especially medicines that may carry a stigma; understandably, some people do not want others to know they are taking medicine such as antidepressants
  - consider that medicines can help all of us at times for many medical conditions, such as an infection or a headache,

and, because depression is a medical condition, medicines may help

  ◇ it is certainly reasonable to keep private that your child is taking an antidepressant; if it is helping your child feel better, this is what is most important

• taking antidepressant medicine only "as needed"

  ◇ some medicines can be taken as needed, whenever the medical condition needs treating, such as a headache or a stuffy nose from a cold

  ◇ other medicines, including antidepressants, are best given on a regular daily basis, and are not effective when only taken as needed

  ◇ although your child may feel that the antidepressant is not needed some days, it is best to take it daily for at least several weeks, and then after 4 to 6 weeks, discuss with your pediatrician whether the medicine is helping and still needed

POTENTIAL FOR INCREASED RISK OF SUICIDE

A controversial area surrounding the use of antidepressant medicines in children, adolescents, and young adults is the potential for an increased risk of suicide. Since 2004, all classes of antidepressants have a required "black box" warning, as mandated by the FDA. A black box warning is the highest level of warning or concern the FDA can require for a medicine. It does not necessarily mean that the medicine definitively produces the adverse effect, but because of the potential seriousness of the adverse effect, the warning is required. The following is the black box antidepressant warning about suicidal thinking and behavior:

> Antidepressants increased the risk of suicidal thoughts and behavior in children, adolescents, and young adults in short-term studies. Short-term studies did not show an increase in the risk of suicidal thoughts and behavior with antidepressants compared to placebo in adults beyond age 24; there was a reduction

in the risk of suicidality with antidepressant use in patients aged 65 and older. In all patients of all ages who are started on antidepressant therapy, monitor closely for worsening of depression and for emergence of suicidal thoughts and behaviors. Advise families and caregivers of the need for close observation and communication with the prescriber.

It is recommended practice to watch for suicidal ideas or actions in *all* children and adolescents, whether they are taking antidepressant medicines or not. Unfortunately, suicidal thinking and behavior are relatively common in adolescence. The Centers for Disease Control and Prevention (CDC), the federal government's primary health agency, reports that 17 percent of adolescents think about suicide in a given year. Fortunately, most of these adolescents do not successfully commit suicide, but about 2,000 adolescents die from suicide each year. In 2014, suicide was the second leading cause of death among adolescents 15 to 19 years of age, with 1,834 suicides occurring in this age group in 2014.

What prompted the FDA to issue this required black box warning for all antidepressant use in children and adolescents? In 2004, the FDA reviewed the results of 24 studies of several different antidepressants including, but not exclusively, SSRI antidepressants, used to treat depression, anxiety, and obsessive-compulsive disorder in children and adults. More than 4,400 children and adults were enrolled in these studies that compared antidepressants to placebos. Overall, the FDA found that more of the study subjects 24 years of age and younger receiving antidepressants spontaneously reported thoughts of suicide or attempted suicide as compared to those taking a placebo. Of the study subjects taking an antidepressant, 4 of 100, or 4 percent, spontaneously reported thinking about suicide or attempted suicide, as compared to 2 of 100, or 2 percent, of the study subjects taking a placebo. There were no completed suicides in these studies.

The black box warning the FDA required for all antidepressant medicines for children and adults 24 years of age and younger is controversial among many pediatric experts. It is important to view this black box warning in light of other information about suicidality (suicidal thinking and behavior) in children and adolescents. Other studies and surveys of adolescents have demonstrated that as many as 50 to 80 percent of adolescents are thinking about suicide when they are first diagnosed with depression, and up to 35 percent have made a previous suicide attempt.

The method of determining how many adolescents had suicidal thoughts is important to consider in weighing the FDA's study review. Suicidal thoughts that were *spontaneously* reported by the study adolescents were evaluated. Many experts believe that using a structured rating scale form to ask adolescents directly about their suicidal thoughts is a more reliable method to assess for suicidal behavior than spontaneous reporting, as was done in the FDA's initial study analysis. In fact, when the FDA re-analyzed those studies that used structured rating scale forms to evaluate suicidal thinking among adolescents taking an antidepressant, they found antidepressant medicine treatment did *not* increase suicidal behavior and thinking. This led some professional medical organizations, such as the American Academy of Child and Adolescent Psychiatry, to not fully agree with the FDA's analysis and assessment about the potential for antidepressants to increase suicidal behavior in adolescents and young adults.

Another group of researchers re-analyzed these initial FDA studies, in addition to several other relevant studies, and found a very small, 0.7 percent, increased risk of suicidal behavior among adolescents taking an antidepressant. Other researchers, using different statistical analytic techniques, evaluated the FDA studies and concluded that antidepressants do *not* increase suicidal behavior in adolescents. Additional important information comes from several different studies that demonstrate that as antidepressant prescribing declines due to fear of increasing suicidal behavior, the rate of adolescent suicide increases. This finding suggests that antidepressant therapy is effective in treating depression, decreasing the likelihood that treated adolescents will attempt suicide. In other words, many experts feel that the risk of not prescribing an antidepressant to depressed adolescents is greater than the risk of increased suicidal behavior, as suggested by some of these studies.

Why do some of the studies suggest an increase in suicidal behavior from antidepressant medicine therapy while other studies point toward a reduced risk of suicidal behavior from antidepressant medicines? The answer has not been clearly determined, although some ideas have been described in published medical journals. Some experts believe that as an antidepressant begins to improve an adolescent's depression, the adolescent may be more likely to talk to someone for the first time about past or present suicidal thoughts. Other experts have suggested that in a small number of depressed adolescents, as antidepressant medicine therapy begins to treat depression, small decreases in inhibitory thought and activity allow enough increased energy to cause underlying suicidal gestures to be noticed.

All experts agree that when an antidepressant medicine is begun for a child, adolescent, or young adult, it is important to carefully monitor for changes in activities or behavior that may indicate an increased risk of suicide. These behaviors and changes include increased restlessness, irritability, or agitation. This watchfulness is most important in the first several weeks of starting an antidepressant. If your child or adolescent is prescribed an antidepressant, your pediatrician will discuss this need for watchfulness with you. It is also important to frequently communicate with your pediatrician during this time, and to attend scheduled follow-up appointments. When antidepressant medicines are effective, benefits noticed first commonly include improvements in sleep and appetite, with improvements in productive thinking and activity following next. Improvements in mood are often not noticeable until 3 to 6 weeks after the antidepressant is begun.

All of the SSRI antidepressants listed above are available in generic form, with the exception of vilazodone (Viibryd). The SSRIs having the most experience of use in children and adolescents, fluoxetine (Prozac) and escitalopram (Lexapro), are available as generic tablets, capsules, and liquids. These generic SSRIs are inexpensive, with a one-month's supply costing as little as $4 at some pharmacies. Most SSRI tablets are "scored," which means each tablet has a line of demarcation in the middle of the tablet, so it can be easily broken into equal half tablets. This scoring helps when smaller doses are needed. Some insurance companies require that half-tablet pieces of higher-strength tablets be given, rather than whole tablets of the prescribed dose, and the scoring on the tablets helps if your insurance company has this requirement. The insurance companies save money by, for example, asking patients to get a 10 mg daily dose by taking one-half of a 20 mg tablet, rather than taking a 10 mg tablet.

St. John's Wort

St. John's wort is a CAM product (complementary and alternative medicine) derived from the plant *Hypericum perforatum*. (See chapter 3 for additional information about CAM products.) St. John's wort has been studied in adults with mild or moderate depression, and some studies have determined that it is an effective antidepressant. However, several larger studies have determined that it is not effective. No studies have been performed in children. None of the studies in adults found St. John's wort to be more effective than SSRI antidepressant medicines. St. John's wort is not recommended in pediatric published treatment guidelines.

As discussed in chapter 3, CAM products are loosely regulated for content and purity and may not contain the active ingredients in the amounts stated on the product bottle or package. Additional studies have shown that St. John's wort can interact with many other medicines, resulting in increased adverse effects from or reduced effectiveness of these medicines. If you are interested in using nonmedicine therapy for your child's depression, psychotherapy (counseling) is more likely to be effective and is safer than St. John's wort. I recommend not using St. John's wort to treat your child's depression until more studies testing its effectiveness and safety in children are conducted and published in medical journals.

Attention Deficit–Hyperactivity Disorder

With 8 percent of children and youth diagnosed with attention deficit–hyperactivity disorder (ADHD), it is the most common neurobehavioral disorder of childhood. ADHD is considered to be a chronic condition; more than half of the people who have ADHD as children will continue to display symptoms into adulthood. Symptoms that define ADHD are described as three main types: inattention, hyperactivity, and impulsivity. ADHD is diagnosed by a pediatrician when these symptoms become noticeable to parents, teachers, and others, as the symptoms become disruptive to the child's normal daily life, including social interactions and school academic performance. Pediatricians use information obtained from parent- and teacher-completed rating scales to diagnose ADHD in a child. The prevalence of ADHD has increased over the past 20 years, although it is not clear whether more children are developing ADHD or recently published, more-inclusive diagnostic criteria is a main reason. Some experts believe that ADHD is diagnosed too easily and frequently by pediatricians and other physicians.

ADHD has been well studied and we have good evidence from many published studies that treatment with medications is effective. Behavioral therapy can be additionally beneficial for some children, especially younger children. The goal of behavioral therapy is to modify a child's physical and social environment to change behavior and manage common symptoms of ADHD. Behavior training techniques can be used by parents at home and teachers in the child's classroom and school environment. These techniques are not as effective as medicine therapy, but the combination of behavior therapy and medicine therapy may allow the child to require less medicine for good control of ADHD symptoms.

Stimulant Medicines

Many clinical studies have evaluated various medicines for ADHD, with these studies providing good evidence that medication therapy successfully manages ADHD symptoms for most children. The most effective class of medicines is stimulants, which includes various formulations and chemical modifications of two stimulant medicines: methylphenidate and amphetamine. It seems paradoxical that stimulant medicines can help control a medical disorder that is characterized in part by increased activity. Although we do not fully understand how stimulant medications improve ADHD symptoms, it is believed that they increase the activity of dopamine in the brain. Dopamine is an important neurotransmitter, a chemical that relays messages between nerve cells in our brains and other parts of our bodies. A main function of dopamine is regulation of the reward-behavior systems of our brains, which control pleasure, learning, and appetite behaviors.

The stimulant medicines methylphenidate and amphetamine are classified as first-line therapy for treating ADHD and are considered very effective, with at least 75 percent of children demonstrating good control of ADHD from a stimulant medicine. Children and adolescents beginning treatment with a stimulant will often notice benefits quickly, within the first 1 or 2 days of treatment. Many different stimulant medication products and formulations are available, which allows pediatricians to choose from a wide variety of options (table 4.1). Stimulants are available as swallow tablets and capsules, capsules that can be opened and sprinkled onto food, chewable and dissolvable tablets, liquids, and a patch formulation that is applied to the skin, similar to a bandage.

An important characteristic of the stimulant medicine products that can be used to individualize therapy for young children, older

Table 4.1. Several stimulant drug products

Stimulant	Product names
methylphenidate	• Ritalin
	• Methylin
	• Metadate
	• Concerta
	• Daytrana (patch)
dexmethylphenidate	• Focalin XR
amphetamine	• Adderall
dextroamphetamine	• Dexedrine
	• Dextrostat
lisdexamfetamine	• Vyvanse

children, and adolescents is duration of effect, or how long the product controls ADHD symptoms. The stimulant medicine products are categorized as short-acting, medium-acting, and long-acting, with durations of 3 to 5 hours, 5 to 8 hours, and 8 to 12 hours, respectively. The medium-acting and long-acting products are especially useful in treating children and adolescents who are in school, because a dose can be given in the morning at home, before school begins, providing benefit for the entire school day. Many adolescents will also take a short-acting stimulant as needed in the early evening to help with homework, studying for exams, or additional work on school assignments.

Unlike SSRI antidepressants (discussed in the previous section), stimulant medicines can be taken as needed, when you and your child believe it is warranted. Most children and adolescents will take their stimulant medicines daily Monday through Friday for school, and depending upon how much schoolwork is assigned for weekends, they may or may not take medicine over the weekend. While stimulant medicines may not be needed on weekends when no studying or other schoolwork is planned, continuing stimulant medicines on weekends has the benefit of improved focus for other important activities, such as driving safely. Many adolescents who work at part-time jobs on weekends and need to concentrate and be attentive at their job take their stimulant medicine as needed prior to going to work.

Nonstimulant Medicines

Several nonstimulant medicines are available to treat ADHD. Although they do not control ADHD as effectively as the stimulant medicines, they can be beneficial and they have a role for some children and adolescents. Nonstimulants can be helpful for children and adolescents who have a contraindication for use of a stimulant (a medical reason for not using), such as a severe tic disorder, or for children who have developed unmanageable adverse effects from a stimulant medicine. The nonstimulant medicines include atomoxetine (Strattera), clonidine (Kapvay), and guanfacine (Intuniv). Clonidine and guanfacine can also be helpful as an additional medication to be taken with a stimulant, especially in children or adolescents who have other medical disorders, such as anxiety or aggression. Because clonidine and guanfacine commonly cause tiredness, they are often given at bedtime, unlike stimulants, which are best given in the morning. Nonstimulants can also be helpful when treating children and adolescents with a history of substance abuse, or when substance abuse is present in close family members, because nonstimulants are not likely to be abused and diverted to others.

ADVERSE EFFECTS OF STIMULANT AND NONSTIMULANT MEDICINES

Stimulant medicines are safe medicines overall and are used by thousands of children and adolescents without problems. Most of the adverse effects from stimulants can be managed without difficulty. Common adverse effects, and methods to manage them, include:

- decreased appetite, weight loss, and abdominal pain
  ◇ give stimulants after breakfast or a snack in the morning; if weight loss occurs, encourage eating bigger meals and more calories in the evening, when the stimulant has worn off
- decreased sleep
  ◇ give long-acting stimulants in the morning, preferably no later than about 10:00
- headaches
  ◇ use acetaminophen (Tylenol) or ibuprofen (Motrin, Advil) as needed; a reduced dose of the stimulant medicine may help lessen the headaches (discuss any adjustments in dose with your pediatrician)

These adverse effects can also be decreased by giving a smaller stimulant dose or changing to a different stimulant product. As with starting any new medicine, it is helpful to frequently communicate with your pediatrician about new adverse effects. Your pediatrician will discuss with you options for managing them.

Some people believe that stimulant medicines may have dangerous adverse effects on a child's or adolescent's heart and blood pressure. This concern has recently been evaluated by several committees of experts, and the available evidence indicates that for a child or adolescent with a healthy cardiovascular system, stimulant medicines do not pose an increased risk. It is expected that the prescribing pediatrician will routinely check your child's blood pressure at each follow-up visit.

Stimulant medicines may also worsen a tic disorder (abnormal repetitive muscle movements or vocal sounds). Most children and adolescents who have a mild tic disorder can still be successfully treated with a stimulant medicine, as the tic disorder will not be noticeably worsened. If it is, atomoxetine (Strattera), a nonstimulant medicine, can be used instead of a stimulant, and is less likely to worsen tic disorders.

Some adolescents will notice that they are "less fun" or less spontaneous in their actions when taking stimulant medicines. This is likely due to the stimulant medicine's controlling impulsivity and hyperactivity, hallmark symptoms of ADHD. While the adolescent's friends may miss the comical behavior, the increased academic performance from the stimulant's beneficial effect is welcomed.

Common adverse effects from the nonstimulant medicines differ from stimulants, mainly for their potential to cause tiredness or sedation, especially with clonidine (Kapvay) and guanfacine (Intuniv). Atomoxetine (Strattera) can decrease appetite and result in weight loss as well, although it is usually not as noticeable as with the stimulant medicines.

BLACK BOX WARNING

Atomoxetine (Strattera) has a black box warning on its prescribing information and labeling, for a potential increase in suicidal thinking and behavior in children and adolescents. As described above in the discussion of depression, suicidal thinking and behavior commonly occur in adolescents overall, even when no medicines are given. In studies of atomoxetine used to allow the FDA to make a decision about approving its use, suicidal thinking and behavior was found to occur slightly more often, 5 of 1,357 study subjects (0.04 percent), as compared to none of the 851 study subjects receiving a placebo. Because of this very small percentage, recommendations include discussing the potential for an increased risk of suicidal thinking and behavior and what symptoms to be watchful for when atomoxetine is begun in an adolescent.

POTENTIAL FOR ABUSE AND DIVERSION OF
STIMULANT MEDICINES

All of the stimulant medicines used to treat ADHD are classified as C-II controlled substances, which limits the amount of medicine the pediatrician can typically prescribe at one time to a 30-day supply with no refills. The reason for this controlled drug classification relates to the significant abuse and diversion potential for the stimulant medicines. Understandably, some parents express concerns about giving a controlled drug with abuse potential to their child or adolescent.

Children and adolescents with ADHD have a higher risk of abusing alcohol and drugs because of underlying ADHD symptoms and traits of the disorder. There is some evidence from studies that this risk is reduced when ADHD is successfully treated with stimulant medicines. There is very little evidence that stimulant medicines are abused or misused by successfully treated adolescents. A greater concern relates to the diversion of stimulant medicines to people who do not have ADHD for abuse and misuse. This is a primary reason for the controlled status of stimulant medicines, to limit the amount of medicine that is potentially available to others for nonmedical and inappropriate use. Surveys of high school and university students indicate that it is relatively easy for students without ADHD to obtain stimulant medicines from friends and family members for use as aids to improve exam scores and study time.

Some parents may have concerns about their child becoming "addicted" to a long-term use of stimulants. This concern is unfounded, as the term *addiction* implies that the person has physical and psychological dependence on the medication, which does not occur with stimulants when given to children and adolescents who have ADHD. Stimulant medicines can be stopped at any time without adverse effects, and it is common to stop the drug on weekends and summers, when school is not in session. The stimulant medicines with a longer duration of effect, such as Vyvanse, Concerta and Focalin XR, are less prone to diversion and abuse, as compared to the pharmaceutical dosage forms with a short duration of effect, such as Ritalin. Due to their pharmaceutical dosage form, the longer-acting dosage forms are not as likely to result in quick, immediate effects when abused and taken by others for whom the medicine was not prescribed.

You and your adolescent can take several measures to decrease the risks of abuse and diversion with stimulant medicines. Perhaps most important is to keep the stimulant medicine container in a safe, nonvisible place at home. I tell university students when they are prescribed a stimulant medicine to keep it out of sight in their dorm room or apartment, to reduce the likelihood that it will be noticed and possibly taken by someone who is visiting. Parents can also carefully monitor the number of tablets or capsules remaining in the stimulant medicine bottle, matching it to the expected number according to the date of when the bottle was obtained at the pharmacy.

CONSIDERATIONS AT THE PHARMACY

There are many different stimulant medicine products pediatricians can choose from to prescribe for your child or adolescent who has ADHD. As discussed above, a main difference among these products is how long they provide a beneficial effect; the time range is large, from 3 to 12 hours. Your pediatrician will discuss with you how long your child's stimulant typically lasts and how many times a day your child or adolescent should be given the medicine.

Most of the brand name stimulant medicines, such as Ritalin, are available as generic dosage forms, and these will be less expensive. Many of the stimulant products can be relatively expensive, however, costing up to several hundred dollars for a 30-day supply. Some of the generic products can be rather expensive as well, although less costly than the equivalent trade name product. The amount you will pay at the pharmacy also depends upon your health insurance coverage, if any, and what medicines your health insurance plan will pay for. Discuss your insurance coverage with your pediatrician when a stimulant is first prescribed or changed, and check with your health insurance provider to verify what stimulant products are covered and at what level.

An additional difference among the stimulant products is how they are taken: some products can be chewed, dissolved in the mouth, sprinkled over soft foods, or taken as a liquid, while other tablet or capsule products must be swallowed whole, and not chewed or crushed. One stimulant product, Concerta, is manufactured with a unique capsule that may pass through your child's intestinal tract without dissolving, and may appear whole and relatively intact in your child's stool. This is normal; the medicine has been absorbed by the body. Be sure to discuss all of these issues with your pharmacist and pediatrician.

Complementary and Alternative Medicine (CAM) Supplements

The CAM product polyunsaturated fatty acids, also called omega-3 fatty acids, has been studied to treat ADHD in children. A recent published analysis of 10 studies including 699 children with ADHD treated with omega-3 fatty acids demonstrated that this supplement can have a small beneficial effect to improve ADHD symptoms. Omega-3 fatty acids have not been directly compared to stimulant or nonstimulant medicines. If you decide to try treating ADHD by giving an omega-3 fatty acid to your child, it is best to use a product with a "USP Verified" stamp or logo on the bottle or package label, indicating that the product is more likely to accurately contain what is stated on the label, without contaminants. See chapter 3 for more information about choosing a CAM supplement product.

If used, an omega-3 fatty acid supplement is probably best added to a stimulant or nonstimulant ADHD medicine. Talk with your pediatrician to let him or her know that you would like to add this supplement to your child's other medication. Parents with concerns about treating ADHD with medication therapy may also consider use of an omega-3 fatty acid supplement product alone, without a stimulant or nonstimulant ADHD medication. Speak with your pediatrician before trying this, however.

Summary Points for Parents

• Depression is common in adolescents.

• Psychotherapy, or counseling, effectively treats mild depression.

- Selective serotonin reuptake inhibitor medicines (SSRIs) effectively treat moderate and severe depression.

- A combination of psychotherapy and SSRIs is more likely to effectively treat moderate to severe depression than either used alone.

- It often takes 4 to 6 weeks for SSRIs to become effective, and they are best used daily, and not occasionally taken "as needed."

- Most adverse effects from use of SSRIs are manageable.

- An increased risk of suicide from use of SSRIs is possible, although this risk is small and largely outweighed by the benefit of medication therapy to treat depression.

- Stimulant medicines effectively treat ADHD symptoms.

- Nonstimulant medicines effectively treat ADHD symptoms, and are best reserved for children unlikely to benefit from a stimulant medicine, because they are not as effective as stimulant medicines.

- Use of stimulant medicines in children and adolescents does not result in "addiction," although these medicines can be abused by others.

5

Vaccines

Vaccines are so important to children's medical care that a book about pediatric health care and medicines would not be complete without a chapter devoted to them. This chapter will review essential information about vaccines—also called immunizations—including how effective they are, why they are necessary, and what safety concerns and other worries many parents have about them. (Many good sources of information about pediatric vaccines discuss vaccines in depth and are listed later in the chapter.)

In recent years, more and more parents have become apprehensive about vaccines. Here are some of the most common questions health care professionals hear. If you have some of these concerns, you are not alone.

- Are all pediatric vaccines still necessary?
- Are vaccines safe?
- Is it harmful to give multiple vaccine shots on the same day, at the same doctor's appointment?

If you have concerns about giving vaccines to your infant or child, your best first step is to discuss the issue with your pediatrician. Tell the pediatrician your specific fears and ask him or her

(*continued on page 110*)

5-1. Recommended Immunization Schedule for Children and Adolescents Aged 18 Ye...

Vaccine	Birth	1 mo	2 mos	4 mos	6 mos	9 mos	1 m...
Hepatitis B[1] (HepB)	1st dose	← 2nd dose →			←		3rd
Rotavirus[2] (RV) RV1 (2-dose series); RV5 (3-dose series)			1st dose	2nd dose	(see FN 2)		
Diphtheria, tetanus, & acellular pertussis[3] (DTaP: <7 yrs)			1st dose	2nd dose	3rd dose		
Haemophilus influenzae type b[4] (Hib)			1st dose	2nd dose	(see FN 4)		← 3rd
Pneumococcal conjugate[5] (PCV13)			1st dose	2nd dose	3rd dose		←
Inactivated poliovirus[6] (IPV: <18 yrs)			1st dose	2nd dose	←		
Influenza[7] (IIV)							
Measles, mumps, rubella[8] (MMR)					(see FN 8)	←	
Varicella[9] (VAR)						←	
Hepatitis A[10] (HepA)						←	2
Meningococcal[11] (Hib-MenCY ≥6 weeks; MenACWY-D ≥9 mos; MenACWY-CRM ≥2 mos)							
Tetanus, diphtheria, & acellular pertussis[12] (Tdap: ≥7 yrs)							
Human papillomavirus[13] (HPV)							
Meningococcal B[11]							
Pneumococcal polysaccharide[5] (PPSV23)							

Range of recommended ages for all children

Range of recommended ages for catch-up immunization

Range of recommended a... for certain high-risk grou...

Source: Based on the chart provided by the US Department of Health and Human Services, Centers fo... Disease Control and Prevention

5 mos	18 mos	19–23 mos	2–3 yrs	4–6 yrs	7–10 yrs	11–12 yrs	13–15 yrs	16 yrs	17–18 yrs

4th dose → 5th dose

(see FN 4) →

→

4th dose

Annual vaccination (IIV) 1 or 2 doses | Annual vaccination (IIV) 1 dose only

2nd dose

2nd dose

(see FN 10) →

(11) 1st dose 2nd dose

Tdap

(see FN 13)

(see FN 11)

(see FN 5)

Range of recommended ages for non-high-risk groups that may receive vaccine, subject to individual clinical decision making ☐ No recommendation

Note: For full information regarding the recommended immunizations, including all footnotes (FN), see https://www.cdc.gov/vaccines/schedules/hcp/imz/child-adolescent.html.

(*continued from page 107*) to talk them through with you. Pediatric health care providers, including your pediatrician, share your wish for children—including your child—to be as healthy as possible. Giving the vaccines recommended in the current pediatric immunization schedule (figure 5.1) is an effective way of keeping infants and children healthy and free from disease.

As has been discussed throughout this book, the benefit of giving a drug to an infant or child should outweigh its risks, or adverse effects. Choosing to give any drug to your child is an important decision that you make as a parent. It is a decision informed by advice and recommendations from your child's pediatrician. Vaccines are also considered drugs. All vaccines have risks, or adverse effects, and benefits. For the vast majority of infants or children, the benefits of vaccines greatly outweigh the risks. These benefits include preventing many potentially deadly infectious diseases, such as polio, measles, meningitis, and pertussis (whooping cough).

Vaccines can cause adverse effects, such as soreness at the injection site or a mild fever, but serious adverse effects are rare. The vast majority of infants and children who receive vaccines have no adverse effects from vaccines, other than perhaps a sore arm or thigh after a shot.

Some infants and children have contraindications to receiving some vaccines—in other words, some children should not receive specific vaccines because the risk of adverse effects is greater in these infants and children than for other children, and the risk may outweigh the benefits of the vaccine. For example, if a child is receiving chemotherapy for leukemia, normally scheduled pediatric vaccines will be deferred for this child until chemotherapy treatments are completed. If your child has a contraindication to a vaccine, your pediatrician will recommend adjusting the vaccine schedule.

The Pediatric Immunization Schedule

Each January a new immunization schedule for infants, children, and adolescents younger than 18 years of age is published by the Centers for Disease Control and Prevention (CDC) and is approved by the American Academy of Pediatrics. The pediatric immunization schedule for 2017 is presented in figure 5.1. In some years the pediatric immunization schedule changes only slightly, with new or different age ranges given for specific vaccines, while in other years new vaccine products are added to the schedule, resulting in significant changes. As you can easily see, the recommended vaccines provide protection from many infectious diseases, which is good. It is far better to prevent a serious disease in your child than to have him or her contract the disease and require treatment.

Benefits of Pediatric Vaccines: Diseases Targeted and Prevented

In 1999, the Centers for Disease Control and Prevention, the federal government's main public health agency, published an article describing the ten greatest public health achievements of the twentieth century. The top ten are:

- improved motor vehicle safety
- safer workplaces
- control of infectious diseases
- decline in deaths from coronary heart disease and stroke
- safer and healthier foods
- healthier mothers and babies
- family planning
- fluoridation of drinking water
- recognition of tobacco use as a health hazard
- vaccination

Considering the good that vaccines have done it is not surprising that vaccination is listed as one of these public health achievements. Pediatric vaccines have prevented literally millions of infant and child deaths from infectious diseases. Vaccines have eliminated smallpox and have controlled polio in the United States (although not in some other places in the world).

Table 5.1. Prevalence of infectious diseases targeted by vaccines (children and adults in United States)

Disease	Yearly rate in the 20th century (before vaccine use)	2013	Percentage decrease
Diphtheria	21,053	0	100
Pertussis (whooping cough)	200,752	24,231	88
Tetanus	580	19	97
Polio	16,316*	0	100
Measles	530,217	184	99.9
Mumps	162,344	438	99.7
Rubella (German measles)	47,745	9	99.9
Haemophilus influenzae type B (meningitis)	20,000	18	99.9

Source: American Academy of Pediatrics *Red Book* (2015)

*1951–1954

Most of the infectious diseases we have vaccines to protect us from—such as measles, pertussis, and mumps—continue to develop in the United States. New outbreaks of measles and pertussis have recently occurred in the United States, in part because unimmunized children spread the viruses and bacteria that cause these illnesses to other susceptible children, including children who are still too young to be immunized against these diseases. Table 5.1 lists several infectious diseases targeted by current pediatric vaccines, showing their prevalence before and after regular vaccine use. The dramatic decline indicates how effective vaccines are. When rates of unimmunized children rise, as has been happening in recent years (for example, fewer children are being vaccinated against measles), so do the rates of, and deaths from, these infectious diseases.

Table 5.2 lists the infectious diseases the current pediatric vaccines target. Most of these infectious diseases are completely averted when a child has received the corresponding vaccine, since the vaccine prompts the immune system to prevent disease when a child is exposed to the virus or bacteria that causes the illness. Some of the other infectious diseases, such as influenza (the flu), may not always be completely prevented in a child who has received the vaccine. However, if the infection occurs in a child who has received the flu vaccine, it is much less likely to lead to a serious illness.

For example, if a child who receives a flu shot is exposed to the flu virus from other children, the child may not become ill at all, or he or she may develop a mild case of flu, perhaps becoming ill for only several days. In a child who has not received a flu shot, it is more likely that he or she will develop more serious illness when exposed to flu viruses. A flu shot may prevent the child from needing hospitalization, which might have been required if the sick child had not been vaccinated. Vaccinations against flu also prevent death in children by minimizing the flu illness. Children die each year from influenza, with as many as 171 children dying during an influenza season in recent years. Many of these children who died did not receive a flu shot, and it is quite likely that their deaths could have been prevented had they received a flu shot.

Adverse Effects from Vaccines

Many parents who are hesitant for their children to receive vaccines have concerns over vaccine safety and the possibility of adverse effects. Similar to other drugs, vaccines undergo many years of phased testing for safety and effectiveness in humans before they are licensed for use and made available to the public. And just like other drugs, vaccines have the potential to produce adverse effects. Fortunately, most adverse effects from vaccines are mild, such as soreness at the site of the injection.

Even after a vaccine has been approved and licensed by the

(*continued on page 116*)

Table 5.2. Diseases that vaccines protect against

Disease	How is the disease spread?	What type of illness can the disease cause?	Is death possible from this disease?
Hepatitis B (virus)	Birth from an infected mother; sex (adolescents); blood from an infected person; intravenous drug use	Hepatitis (liver disease)	Yes
Rotavirus (virus)	Contact with stool from an infected person	Diarrhea and dehydration	Yes
Diphtheria (bacteria)	Respiratory (coughing, sneezing, contact with nose, mouth)	Fever; sore throat; difficulty breathing	Yes
Tetanus (lockjaw) (bacteria)	Found in the soil and dirty areas and infects an open wound	Lockjaw; severe muscle spasms	Yes
Pertussis (whooping cough) (bacteria)	Respiratory (coughing, sneezing, contact with nose, mouth)	Cough; pneumonia	Yes
Haemophilus influenzae type b (bacteria)	Respiratory (coughing, sneezing, contact with nose, mouth)	Meningitis; pneumonia	Yes
Pneumococcal (bacteria)	Respiratory (coughing, sneezing, contact with nose, mouth)	Meningitis; pneumonia; ear infections	Yes
Polio (virus)	Contact with stool from an infected person	Muscle paralysis	Yes
Influenza (the flu) (virus)	Respiratory (coughing, sneezing, contact with nose, mouth)	Fever; cough; ear infections; muscle aches; headache; vomiting; pneumonia	Yes

Disease	How is the disease spread?	What type of illness can the disease cause?	Is death possible from this disease?
Measles (virus)	Respiratory (coughing, sneezing, contact with nose, mouth)	Fever; cough; rash; pneumonia	Yes
Mumps (virus)	Respiratory (coughing, sneezing, contact with nose, mouth)	Swelling of salivary glands; fever; muscle aches	Yes, but rare and mostly in adults
Rubella (German measles) (virus)	Respiratory (coughing, sneezing, contact with nose, mouth)	Fever; rash— usually mild in children, but causes many birth defects if mother develops disease while pregnant	Most dangerous to a fetus (before birth)
Varicella (chicken pox) (virus)	Respiratory (coughing, sneezing, contact with nose, mouth)	Rash; skin infections; pneumonia; swelling of the brain	Yes
Hepatitis A (virus)	Contact with stool from an infected person	Fever; nausea; tiredness; jaundice	Yes
Meningo-coccal (bacteria)	Respiratory (coughing, sneezing, contact with nose, mouth)	Meningitis; severe whole body infection	Yes
Human papillomavirus (HPV) (virus)	Skin-to-skin contact, usually through sexual activity	Genital cancers of both sexes, including cervical cancer in females, and genital warts in both sexes	Yes (due to cancer development)

(*continued from page 113*) FDA, it continues to be monitored for safety concerns and rare adverse effects. These safety monitoring systems and programs include the Vaccine Adverse Event Reporting System, the Vaccine Safety Datalink, the Post-Licensure Rapid Immunization Safety Monitoring System, and the Clinical Immunization Safety Assessment Project. The FDA and the CDC recognize the public's concern about vaccine safety and have established these monitoring programs to keep a watchful eye and respond quickly to any safety issues.

In addition, various groups of pediatric medical experts, such as those at the Institute of Medicine, have reviewed all of the safety and epidemiologic data about vaccines and their potential adverse effects and have published their findings. These reports have been summarized in nontechnical language for the public and can easily be found on various Internet sites (see table 5.3 for more information). One of the best Internet sites for parents is from the CDC, available at www.cdc.gov/vaccines. One very important finding from these vaccine safety reviews is that there is no credible evidence that the MMR vaccine is a cause of autism. Much information and many studies have been evaluated by groups of various scientific experts, and all of this information points to no link between the MMR vaccine and autism.

Common Myths about Vaccines

Here are three common myths about vaccines and information that reveals the myths for what they are—myths, not truth.

MYTH: Administering more than one vaccine at one time overloads or weakens the immune system.
FACTS: Our immune systems are exposed to many viruses and bacteria from other people and the environment every day, and have evolved for this purpose. Most vaccines include several of the most important parts, termed antigenic components, of the

viral or bacterial causes of the targeted infectious diseases, and can easily be "handled" by our immune systems to provide protection.

MYTH: Most vaccines are no longer needed, as these infections no longer occur.
FACTS: Of all the diseases for which vaccines have been developed, only smallpox has been eradicated and is no longer a threat to the public. Although wild polio has not been contracted in the United States in many years, the viruses that cause polio still exist naturally in other parts of the world and can be brought into the United States by others who have traveled outside of the country. All of the infectious diseases listed in table 5. 2 continue to be a threat and can be contracted and cause disease in your child.

MYTH: Vaccine doses can be separated, and spread out, and given at different times instead of on the timetable that is recommended by the pediatric immunization schedule.
FACTS: The current pediatric immunization schedule includes vaccine doses administered at specific times, often requiring more than one dose of each vaccine given at different times. The recommended separation times between each vaccine dose have been clinically tested and shown to be the most effective intervals. Vaccine dose separation times greater than recommended in the pediatric immunization schedule have not been tested and may cause vaccines to be less effective and therefore increase risk to your child.

Why Some Parents Refuse Vaccines for Their Children

Increasing numbers of parents are refusing one or more of the recommended vaccines for their children. A small minority of parents, about 3 percent, have reported in recent surveys that they refused all vaccines for their children. The most common reasons parents give for refusing vaccines include the belief that vaccines are no longer needed and worries about vaccine adverse effects. Other concerns expressed by parents include the belief that "natural" infection is better than vaccine-induced immunity, the conviction that vaccines are not effective, or fears about vaccine additives, such as aluminum. Other parents believe in freedom of choice and object to mandated requirements of vaccine administration for their children. If you have one or more of these concerns about vaccines for your children, you need to discuss these concerns with your pediatrician. Your pediatrician, like you, wants your children to be as healthy as possible and likely will be glad to discuss these issues with you.

Good Information Sources about Vaccines

Unfortunately, many Internet sites about vaccines do not provide scientifically and medically accurate information. Some of these sites may scare you about vaccines and make you afraid for your children to be immunized. Table 5.3 lists scientifically and medically accurate Internet websites that are reliable and that have been prepared by medical professionals. I encourage you to review the information on your own time. One especially compelling site is www.immunize.org/reports. This site, from the Immunization Action Coalition, includes true accounts of children and adults who have suffered or died from vaccine-preventable diseases. If you have concerns or doubts that vaccines are no longer needed, this website will provide you with plenty to think about.

Reducing Pain from Vaccine Shots

Parent surveys indicate that they worry about pain from vaccine shots. This pain can be minimized by using several methods, whose effectiveness is supported by published studies. A recently published review of these approaches found scientific evidence that the following approaches can decrease pain and discomfort in infants and children associated with vaccine shots:

Table 5.3. Internet sites with reliable vaccine information

Internet site	Organization
www.vaccineinformation.org	Immunization Action Coalition
www.immunize.org/reports	Real-life accounts of children who suffered or died from vaccine-preventable diseases, from the Immunization Action Coalition
www.cdc.gov/vaccines	Centers for Disease Control and Prevention
www.healthychildren.org (use the "immunizations" link)	American Academy of Pediatrics
www.pkids.org	Parents of Kids with Infectious Diseases
www.vaccinesafety.org	Institute for Vaccine Safety, Johns Hopkins Bloomberg School of Public Health
www.chop.edu/centers-programs /vaccine-education-center	Vaccine Education Center, Children's Hospital of Philadelphia
www.ecbt.org	Every Child by Two, Carter/ Bumpers Champions for Immunization

- Methods pediatricians and nurses can use:
  - ◇ Administer a sweet-tasting solution of sugar water to infants up to 12 months of age one to two minutes prior to the vaccine injection, using an oral syringe or pacifier.
  - ◇ Have the child sit in the parent's lap for the injection, or use another position that is comfortable to parent and child.

Avoid administering the vaccine to a child who is lying down.
  - ◊ If more than one vaccine is administered at a clinic visit, administer the potentially more painful vaccines, such as MMR, last.
- ◆ Methods you can use as a parent:
  - ◊ Learn distraction techniques that can be used while the shot is administered. Some of the techniques require a little training by your pediatrician's office, so ask your health care provider about these methods in advance.
  - ◊ Consider using an anesthetic cream or ointment on your child's skin where the vaccine shot will likely be given. It is usually best to apply the ointment 30 to 60 minutes prior to the vaccine shot (usually while you and your child are still at home). These creams include lidocaine/prilocaine (EMLA), a prescription drug, or lidocaine 4 percent (LMX 4), available as an over-the-counter drug product. It is important to place these creams on the appropriate areas where the vaccines will be given, and in a specific manner— your pediatrician's office will explain this to you.
  - ◊ Breastfeed your infant to decrease vaccine shot pain. Begin nursing prior to the shot and continue for several minutes afterwards.
  - ◊ For children 3 years age or older, use blowing exercises, such as blowing bubbles, party blowers, or pinwheels during vaccine administration.

Vaccines and My Family

Because I believe vaccines are an effective means to prevent or minimize many dangerous infectious diseases, my own two nearly adult children, my wife, and I have received all of the recommended vaccines for our ages. We have flu shots each year, and both my son and my daughter have received the human papillomavirus (HPV) vaccine.

Summary Points for Parents

- Pediatric vaccines are one of the most effective means to prevent serious diseases in infants, children, and adolescents, and are life-saving medicines.

- Overall, pediatric vaccine products are safe, and they are continuously monitored for new safety concerns.

- Pediatric vaccines can have adverse effects, but the vast majority are mild.

- Some infants and children, a relatively small number, should not receive some pediatric vaccines, as they can cause serious adverse effects.

- The current pediatric immunizations schedule is best followed as recommended and not delayed or adapted to alternative schedules.

- Some parents have concerns about pediatric vaccines, and these concerns are best discussed with their pediatrician.

- Several reliable and medically accurate Internet websites can be viewed by parents for more information.

- Several effective methods can be used by you and your pediatrician to reduce pain from vaccine shots.

6

Getting Reliable Information about Medicines

The Internet and Your Pharmacist

This chapter will help you find reliable information about pediatric medicines and diseases on the Internet. It will also describe how your pharmacist can answer your questions and provide information you need about medications.

The Internet

The Internet can be a source of highly accurate and useful information. Unfortunately, because nearly anyone can set up a website and place information on the Internet, there is a great deal of inaccurate and misleading information on the Internet as well. The information on Internet sites may not be medically accurate or it may be biased for a specific cause or purpose, such as promoting antivaccine views or specific supplement products. Below I offer some guidance to help you determine whether a specific website is likely to be reliable and a good source of information.

Published surveys of the American public indicate that many adults search the Internet for information about health, including diseases and medications and other treatments. Studies by researchers about commonly visited Internet websites indicate that many of the top websites identified by common search engines, such as Wikipedia, often miss much valuable information about health topics, and thus can easily be misleading to readers. Listed in table 6.1 are characteristics to consider when reading a specific Internet site about health and medicines and other medical treatments.

Pay attention to the main intent of the site. Ask yourself if the primary purpose of the site is to inform and educate you about the disease and its medical therapies, or if it is mainly intended to promote a specific drug or cause. Websites with the broader purpose of educating the public are generally more informative and likely to provide you with useful information, as they are usually developed by nonprofit medical organizations (web addresses ending in .org), educational institutions (ending in .edu), or governmental agencies (ending in .gov). Websites developed by commercial institutions (ending in .com), have a primary purpose to sell something, such as a drug, and are more likely to include misleading information, or information that is not complete. While some websites ending in .com, such as a website for a specific trade name drug product, may provide some useful information, it is important to recognize that the primary purpose of a .com site is to sell. Internet sites from educational or medical organizations are more likely to provide complete and less biased information about all drugs, not just one drug, that can be used treat a specific illness.

Throughout this book I have referred to specific organizations or government health agencies that sponsor reliable and medically accurate websites. These organizations and agencies include the Food and Drug Administration (www.fda.gov/drugs), the Centers for Disease Control and Prevention (www.cdc.gov and www.cdc .gov/vaccines), and the American Academy of Pediatrics (www.aap .org and www.healthychildren.org). Other reliable and medically accurate websites are listed in table 6.2.

Table 6.1. Finding reliable information: what to look for in a website

What to look for	Meaning
About Us / About This Site	• What is the purpose of the website—is it to educate and inform you, or to sell you a product? • Does the website have a board of directors with names listed? Are the listed names qualified health care professionals?
Website ending in ".org," ".edu," or ".gov"	Websites ending with these abbreviations are more likely to provide accurate medical information: • ".org" = organization, such as a professional medical organization • ".edu" = educational institution, such as a university • ".gov" = government, such as the federal government health agencies
Contact Us / Ask A Question	• You should be able to contact someone at the website or ask a question
Website ending in ".com"	• ".com" = Commercial site • Information provided is more likely to be biased and incomplete
Last Updated	• Medical information changes rapidly. Look for a website that has been updated within the past 6–12 months

What to look for	Meaning
Advertisements labeled	• Advertisements should be clearly labeled as advertisements
Privacy Statement	• If personal information is requested, the website should have a policy on how this information will be used or shared
References or Links to Additional Information, or "Source"	• Medical facts and claims should be supported by published studies or other reliable websites, as a reference or source
Search	• Searching within a website allows you to find more information

Your Pharmacist

Your pharmacist can be one of the best sources of information about your child's medicines. Not only is your pharmacist knowledgeable about medicines, but he or she is also usually readily available to answer questions. Unlike physicians, pharmacists are available without an appointment. It may be difficult for the pharmacist to find time for questions when the pharmacy is busy, so plan your visit for a less busy time. The busiest times in community pharmacies are usually early morning, later afternoon (when many people go to and from work), Mondays and Fridays, and before holidays. A good time to call or visit your pharmacist with a question is midweek and midafternoon. Some pharmacies are open 24 hours a day, so you can call any time at these pharmacies.

Try to get to know one or two pharmacists at the pharmacy you use. If you develop a comfortable patient-pharmacist relationship

Table 6.2. Medically accurate Internet sites for health information

Site	Sponsor and information provided
www.fda.gov/drugs	• Food and Drug Administration • much valuable information, including the link "Information for Consumers"
www.cdc.gov	• Centers for Disease Control and Prevention • health information on a wide variety of topics, including diseases and treatment, traveling outside the US, and much more • www.cdc.gov/vaccines provides specific information about vaccines
www.healthychildren.org	• American Academy of Pediatrics • wide variety of health topics about infants, children, and adolescents
www.kidshealth.org	• Nemours Center for Health Media • wide variety of pediatric health information written specifically for parents, children, and adolescents
www.nlm.nih.gov/ medlineplus	• US National Library of Medicine, National Institutes of Health • information on diseases, drugs, medical dictionary, health videos • information in multiple languages
https://ods.od.nih.gov	• National Institutes of Health, Office of Dietary Supplements • information specific for dietary supplements

Site	Sponsor and information provided
www.safemedication.com	• American Society of Health-System Pharmacists
	• includes unique useful information about medicines for children and adults, such as How to Administer Medicines (e.g., into ears, nose), how to reduce drug costs, and others

with one or two pharmacists, you may feel more comfortable asking questions. Just as things go better when you like your doctor and dentist, you will feel more comfortable if you like your pharmacist. If you don't like the pharmacists at your current pharmacy, find another pharmacy where you feel more comfortable.

It is best to use only one pharmacy for your child's and family's medicines. That way the pharmacy will have a list of your current medicines and the pharmacists can warn you if any dangerous drug interactions will occur with new medicines. If you use more than one pharmacy, the other pharmacy may not be aware of what other medicines you or your child are taking, and you may forget to tell them.

Here are good questions to ask your pharmacist about new medicines for your child:

- What is the trade name and generic name of the medicine?
- How is it given? How many times each day? Does it matter what time of day the medicine is given?
- What should I do if I forget, or miss, a dose of this medicine for my child?
- Is this a medicine to give on a regular schedule or only when needed?

- If the medicine is a liquid, how does it taste? Can it be flavored to taste better?
- If the medicine is a tablet or capsule, can it be broken, crushed, or mixed with food?
- Where should I store this medicine: in the refrigerator or at room temperature?
- Should it be given with or without food, or is this not important?
- When will the medicine begin to help my child?
- How will I know if the medicine is helping my child? What should I look for?
- What are the most common side effects? What can I do to lessen the risk of these side effects?
- Is a generic form of the medicine available?
- Does this medicine have refills?
- Is there anything special my child should not do, or be careful doing, when taking this medicine, such as driving (for an adolescent)?
- If my child is taking other medicines, does this medicine interact with or affect any of the other medicines?

I have spoken with many parents who can't remember the names of the medicines their children take. To avoid this situation, it's wise to carry a list of your children's medicines in your wallet or purse, or on your cell phone. On this list write each medicine's name, strength (such as milligrams, mgs), and how many times each day it is given. This information can be especially useful if you are traveling or if you change physicians or move to another area, because your child's medical records may take some time to obtain or transfer.

Summary Points for Parents

- The Internet contains a vast amount of information about health, medicines, and treatments for diseases.

- Much information on the Internet is medically inaccurate or incomplete, and thus misleading.

- Several medically accurate Internet sites are available for the public, written in nontechnical and nonmedical language, and these sites can provide you with reliable information about pediatric medicines and illnesses.

- Your pharmacist can assist you in numerous ways to ensure that medicines are used safely and appropriately for your children.

Maternal Medications
and Breastfeeding

The American Academy of Pediatrics recommends that women breastfeed their newborn infants, when possible, because breastfeeding provides many benefits to the feeding infant and the mother. Human breast milk contains an excellent balance of nutrients and provides additional benefits to the infant, including protection from many types of infection, such as ear infections, diarrhea, and meningitis. Breast milk contains natural antibodies from the mother that decrease the risk of these infections to the infant, and possibly other types of infections as well. Breastfeeding also plays a role in decreasing the risk of sudden infant death syndrome (SIDS) and may decrease the risk of your infant's developing allergies or asthma.

Breastfeeding additionally benefits the mother. The hormones prolactin and oxytocin are released during breastfeeding. These hormones provide a natural feeling of maternal relaxation and maternal-infant bonding and help the mother's body recover and heal from pregnancy and childbirth. Prolactin and oxytocin also delay the return of a mother's menstrual period and decrease a risk of ovarian and breast cancer later in the mother's life.

Most medicines are safe to use while breastfeeding, because the amount of medicine that distributes into breast milk is a small and clinically insignificant amount and is unlikely to be of danger to a feeding infant. However, some medicines do distribute into breast milk to a greater extent and may be of potential concern for the baby's health. For some medicines, especially newer medicines, we do not have enough information to assess if a mother's use of the medicine is clinically significant for her baby's health.

You can search a medically accurate and reliable Internet site called LactMed at http://toxnet.nlm.nih.gov to find information about a specific medicine's use while breastfeeding. This Internet site, from the National Institutes of Health, is updated monthly and is the largest online source of information about maternal medicine use and breastfeeding. It is easy to search for specific medicines and what is known about their effects on an infant.

The amount of a medication that distributes into breast milk depends upon several factors, including how much medication is absorbed by the mother, how the mother metabolizes the medication, chemical characteristics of the medication, the amount of breast milk taken by the infant, the age of the infant, and other factors. The type of medicine (that is, how it functions in the body) and its adverse effect profile are important as well. An additional consideration when thinking about taking medicines while breastfeeding is the effect of the medication on milk production, because some medications can reduce the amount of milk the mother produces.

Many medicines can be safely taken by a woman while breastfeeding her infant. Commonly used medicines considered safe while nursing include the following, which are only several examples of medicines considered safe to use while breastfeeding:

- acetaminophen (Tylenol and generic)
- ibuprofen (Motrin, Advil, and generic)
- loratadine (Claritin and generic)
- cetirizine (Zyrtec and generic)

As with all medicines taken by a mother who is breastfeeding her infant, it is best to use the medicine at the smallest dose possible to control the illness or symptoms, and to take the medicine for the shortest time period possible.

To minimize the amount of medicine that distributes into breast milk consider following these suggestions:

- Take the medicine at a time when you are not as likely to be breastfeeding your infant. For example, take your medicine just after you have breastfed your infant or when you expect your infant to sleep for several hours. This allows the medicine to reach its highest concentration in your blood and milk when your infant will not be breastfeeding.
- Use "short-acting" medicines when possible. Some medicine products are made to last longer, so they can be taken only once or twice per day. Many of these medicines are also available as short-acting products, which means that they often need to be taken three or more times per day. These short-acting products don't stay in the bloodstream as long, which is preferred when you are breastfeeding.
- Always closely watch your infant for any change in behavior if you are taking medicine and breastfeeding. For example, if your infant is sleeping much more, or less, since you started taking a medicine, it is possible that some of the medicine is getting into your milk and affecting your infant.

Some antidepressant medicines, such as the selective serotonin reuptake inhibitors (SSRIs) discussed in chapter 4, are commonly used by adults and deserve careful consideration if a mother would like to breastfeed her infant. Some SSRI medicines may distribute into breast milk to a clinically significant amount and may produce adverse effects in the infant. Although some information is known about antidepressant medicines distributing into breast milk, the long-term effects on an infant's development are still unknown. Many antidepressant medications and similar medications used to treat anxiety or mood disorders distribute into breast milk to some extent, although we do not know how much for many medications. Case reports have been published documenting blood levels of some antidepressants, such as fluoxetine (Prozac and generic), distributing from swallowed breast milk into infants' blood to about 10 percent of the blood level of the mother. This amount may be clinically significant and may result in adverse effects in the infant. The long-term effects of these medications on the developing brain chemistry of infants are unknown.

Concerns have additionally been raised about the use of several herbal products during breastfeeding, including echinacea and St. John's wort. Current recommendations are to avoid these herbal products and possibly other herbal products during breastfeeding. Very little information is known about the use of herbal products by a mother while breastfeeding.

If you desire to breastfeed your infant and you are taking any medicines, including over-the-counter products and herbal products, it is best to inform your pediatrician and discuss the safety of using these medicines while breastfeeding and the potential for adverse effects in your infant.

Giving Medicine in Your Child's Nose, Ear, and Eye

Always wash your hands before and after giving medicine to your child.

Giving Medicine in Your Child's Nose
Liquid Nose Drops

1. You may have to shake the bottle first; check the label.
2. It's best to clear your child's nose before administering the drops. For an infant, use a bulb syringe and suck out the mucus. Have an older child blow his or her nose using a tissue.
3. If the medicine is stored in the refrigerator, warm it up first by holding the bottle and rolling it in your hands for a few minutes.

   For an infant, hold your child as he or she is lying down with the head tilted back a little bit. For an older child, have him or her lie down and tilt the head back a little bit as well. A pillow may help for positioning an older child (place the pillow under the child's upper back, so the head can tilt over the pillow).
4. With the medicine in the dropper, place the dropper just slightly into the nostril. Try not to touch the nostril with the

dropper, although it may be difficult to avoid doing so. Place the medicine drops into the nostril or nostrils as prescribed or recommended.

5. Keep your infant or child lying down for one or two minutes after putting the drops in. An older child may tell you that he or she can taste the medicine in the throat. This is normal. If he or she feels like spitting because of the taste, this is not a problem and you can allow the child to spit.

Giving Medicine in Your Child's Ear
Liquid Ear Drops

1. You may have to shake the bottle first; check the label.
2. If the medicine is stored in the refrigerator, warm it up first by holding the bottle and rolling it in your hands for a few minutes.
3. Place your child on his or her side, with the ear facing up.
4. For younger children (younger than 3 years), gently pull the ear lobe back and down. For older children (3 years and older), gently pull the upper ear lobe back and up.
5. Place the medicine from the dropper into the ear canal. Try not to touch the ear with the dropper.
6. Keep your child lying in this position for about two minutes. You can place a cotton plug into the ear to help keep the medicine in place if your child will not stay still.

Giving Medicine in Your Child's Eye
Liquid Eye Drops

1. You may have to shake the bottle first; check the label.
2. If the medicine is stored in the refrigerator, warm it up first by holding the bottle and rolling it in your hands for a few minutes.
3. Lay your younger child down. Using a warm, moist

washcloth or cotton ball, gently wipe and clean the eyes. An older child can stand up for this part.

4. Gently pull the lower eyelid down until you see a small pouch. Without touching the medicine dropper to the eye, place the liquid drop into this pouch. If the directions are for more than one drop per eye, wait about one minute before putting in the next drop.

5. An older child can stand and tilt the head back. Ask your child to look straight up and then you will gently pull the lower eyelid down until you see a small pouch. Without touching the medicine dropper to the eye, place the liquid drop into this pouch. If the directions are for more than one drop per eye, wait about one minute before putting in the next drop.

6. Try to keep your younger child lying down for a few minutes after putting the eye drops in or have your older child close the eyes for about a minute.

Eye Ointment

1. For eye ointments, use the same directions as above.

2. Gently pull down the lower eyelid until you see a pouch, and then place a line of the ointment medicine into the length of this pouch. Try not to touch the tip of the ointment tube to the eye. Gently move or jiggle the ointment tube as you are nearly done, so the ointment will drop off the end of the tube.

3. Try to keep your child lying down for a few minutes after putting in the ointment, or have your older child close the eyes for about a minute.

References

1. The Science of Medicines for Children

E.A. Bell and D.E. Tunkel, "Over-the-counter cough and cold medications in children: Are they helpful?" *Otolaryngology–Head and Neck Surgery* 142, no. 5 (May 2010): 647–50.

Committee on Drugs, American Academy of Pediatrics, "Off-label use of drugs in children," *Pediatrics* 133, no. 6 (2014): 563–67.

G.L. Kearns, S.M. Abdel-Rahman, S.W. Alander, et al., "Developmental pharmacology—drug disposition, action, and therapy in infants and children," *New England Journal of Medicine* 349, no. 12 (2003): 1157–67.

G.T. Wharton, M.D. Murphy, D. Avant, et al., "Impact of pediatric exclusivity on drug labeling and demonstrations of efficacy," *Pediatrics* 134, no. 2 (August 2014): e512–18.

2. The Art and Practicality of Giving Medicine to Children

L.C. Burghardt, J.W. Ayers, J.S. Brownstein, et al., "Adult prescription drug use and pediatric medication exposures and poisonings," *Pediatrics* 132, no. 1 (2013): 18–27.

Committee on Drugs, American Academy of Pediatrics, "Metric units and the preferred dosing of orally administered liquid medications, *Pediatrics* 135, no. 4 (2015): 784–87.

D. Matsui, "Current issues in pediatric medication adherence," *Pediatric Drugs* 9, no. 5 (2007): 283–88.

M.E. McGrady and K.A. Hommel, "Medication adherence and health care utilization in pediatric chronic illness: A systematic review," *Pediatrics* 132, no. 4 (2013): 730–40.

A. Patel, L. Jacobsen, R. Jhaveri, K.K. Bradford. "Effectiveness of pediatric pill swallowing interventions: A systematic review," *Pediatrics* 135, no. 5 (2015): 883–89.

N. Shehab, P.R. Patel, A. Srinivasan, and D.S. Budnitz, "Emergency department visits for antibiotic-associated adverse events," *Clinical Infectious Diseases* 47 (2008): 735–43.

M.D. Smith, H.A. Spiller, M.J. Casavant, et al., "Out-of-hospital medication errors among young children in the United States, 2002–2012," *Pediatrics* 134, no. 5 (2014): 867–76.

P. Sobhani, J. Christopherson, P.J. Ambrose, R.L. Corelli, "Accuracy of oral liquid measuring devices: A comparison of dosing cup and oral dosing syringe," *The Annals of Pharmacotherapy* 42 (2008): 46–52.

H.S. Yin, B.P. Dreyer, D.C. Ugboaja, et al., "Unit of measurement used and parent medication dosing errors," *Pediatrics* 134, no. 2 (2014): 1–8.

H.S. Yin, A.L. Mendelsohn, M.S. Wolf, et al., "Parents' medication administration errors," *Archives of Pediatrics and Adolescent Medicine* 164, no. 2 (2010): 181–86.

H.S. Yin, R.M. Parker, L.M. Sanders, et al., "Liquid medication errors and dosing tools: A randomized controlled experiment," *Pediatrics* 138, no. 4 (2016): e20160357.

P.J. Zed, C. Haughn, K.J. Black, et al., "Medication-related emergency department visits and hospital admissions in pediatric patients: A qualitative systematic review," *The Journal of Pediatrics* 163 (2013): 477–83.

3. Over-the-Counter, Herbal, Supplement, and Vitamin Products

E.A. Bell and D.E. Tunkel, "Over-the-counter cough and cold medications in children: Are they helpful?" *Otolaryngology-Head and Neck Surgery* 142, no. 5 (2010): 647–50.

L.I. Black, T.C. Clarke, P.M. Barnes, et al., "Use of complementary health approaches among children aged 4–17 years in the United States: National health interview survey, 2007–2012," *National Health Statistics Reports* 78 (2015): 1–18.

Committee on Drugs, American Academy of Pediatrics, "Use of codeine- and dextromethorphan-containing cough remedies in children," *Pediatrics* 99, no. 6 (1997): 918–20.

R.C. Dart, I.M. Paul, G.R. Bond, et al., "Pediatric fatalities associated with over the counter (nonprescription) cough and cold medications," *Annals of Emergency Medicine* 54, no. 4 (2009): 411–17.

N.H. Golden and S.A. Abrams, "Optimizing bone health in children and adolescents," *Pediatrics* 134, no. 4 (2014): e1229–43.

K.J. Kemper, S. Vohra, and R. Walls, "The use of complementary and alternative medicine in pediatrics," *Pediatrics* 122, no. 6 (2008): 1374–86.

Section on Clinical Pharmacology and Therapeutics and Committee on Drugs,

American Academy of Pediatrics, "Clinical report—fever and antipyretic use in children," *Pediatrics* 127, no. 3 (2011): 580–87.

J.M. Sharfstein, M. North, and J.R. Serwint, "Over the counter but no longer under the radar—pediatric cough and cold medications," *New England Journal of Medicine* 357, no. 23 (2007): 2321–24.

H. Szajewska, "What are the indications for using probiotics in children?" *Archives of Disease in Childhood* 101 (2016): 398–403.

D.W. Thomas and F.R. Greer, "Clinical report—probiotics and prebiotics in pediatrics," *Pediatrics* 126, no. 6 (2010): 1217–31.

J.D. Tobias, T.P. Green, and C.J. Cote, "Codeine: Time to say 'no,'" *Pediatrics* 138, no. 4 (2016): e2396–2403.

H.S. Yin, M.S. Wolf, B.P. Dreyer, et al., "Evaluation of consistency in dosing directions and measuring devices for pediatric nonprescription liquid medications," *Journal of the American Medical Association* 304, no. 23 (2010): 2595–2602.

4. Medicines Used to Treat Depression and Attention Deficit–Hyperactivity Disorder

Subcommittee on attention-deficit/hyperactivity disorder, steering committee on quality improvement and management, American Academy of Pediatrics, "ADHD: clinical practice guideline for the diagnosis, evaluation, and treatment of attention-deficit/hyperactivity disorder in children and adolescents," *Pediatrics* 128, no. 5 (2011): 1007–20.

B. Birmaher and D. Brent, "Practice parameter for the assessment and treatment of children and adolescents with depressive disorders," *Journal of the American Academy of Child and Adolescent Psychiatry* 46, no. 11 (2007): 1503–26.

M.H. Bloch and A. Qawasmi, "Omega-3 fatty acid supplementation for the treatment of children with attention-deficit/hyperactivity disorder symptomology: Systematic review with meta-analysis," *Journal of the American Academy of Child and Adolescent Psychiatry* 50, no. 10 (2011): 991–1000.

A.H. Cheung, R.A. Zuckerbrot, P.S. Jensen, et al., "Guidelines for adolescent depression in primary care (GLAD-PC): II. Treatment and ongoing management," *Pediatrics* 120, no. 5 (2007): e1313–26.

S. Cortese, M. Holtman, T. Banaschewski, et al., "Practitioner review: Current best practice in the management of adverse events during treatment with ADHD medications in children and adolescents," *Journal of Child Psychology and Psychiatry* 54, no. 3 (2013): 227–46.

E. Harstad and S. Levy, "Attention-deficit/hyperactivity disorder and substance abuse," *Pediatrics* 134, no. 1 (2014): e293–301.

B. Shain, Committee on adolescence, American Academy of Pediatrics, "Suicide and suicide attempts in adolescents," *Pediatrics* 138, no. 1 (2016): e1–11.

C. Southammakosane and K. Schmitz, "Pediatric psychopharmacology for treatment of ADHD, depression, and anxiety," *Pediatrics* 136, no. 2 (2015): 351–59.

5. Vaccines

K.M. Edwards and J.M. Hackell, "Countering vaccine hesitancy," *Pediatrics* 138, no. 3 (2016): e1–14.

M.A. Maglione, L. Das, L. Raaen, et al., "Safety of vaccines used for routine immunization of US children: A systematic review," *Pediatrics* 134, no. 2 (2014): 1–1.

A. Taddio, M. Appleton, R. Bortolussi, et al., "Reducing the pain of childhood vaccination: An evidence-based clinical practice guideline," *Canadian Medical Journal* 182, no. 18 (2010): e843–55.

Appendix A. Maternal Medications
and Breastfeeding

H.C. Sachs, "The transfer of drugs and therapeutics into human breast milk: An update on selected topics," *Pediatrics* 132, no. 3 (2013): e796–809.

Index

Rocephin (antibiotic), 10

school and daycare, giving medicine during, 35
selective serotonin reuptake inhibitors (SSRIs), for depression, 87–92, 133–34
skin, of infants and children, 8–9
stimulant medicines: and ADHD, 98–100; and considerations at pharmacy, 104–5
St. John's Wort, 96–97
storage of medicines, 19
Strattera, for ADHD, 100
suicide from antidepressant medicines, 92–95
sulfanilamide (antibiotic), 7
supplement products, 71
swallowing medicine, 32–33

tablets and capsules: administering, 32–34; breaking or crushing, 32–34; sprinkle, 33

taste of liquid medicines, 27–31; improving, 28–30
testing medicines in children, 2–7
tetracycline (antibiotic), 13
thalidomide, 7
therapeutic orphan, 1
toxicity, 23
trade vs. generic brands, 18

vaccines: adverse effects of, 110, 113–16; benefits of, 111–13; infectious diseases targeted by, 112, 114–15; information sources about, 118–19; myths about, 116–18; reducing pain from injection sites, 118–20
vitamin D, 79–80
vitamins, 78–80
vomiting after taking medicine, 34

weight, of child, 16